A Dialogue on Ethical Issues of Life and Death

Rocco J. Gennaro

University Press of America,® Inc.
Lanham · New York · Oxford

4720 Boston Way
Lanham, Maryland 20706
UPA Acquisitions Department (301) 459-3366

12 Hid's Copse Rd.
Cumnor Hill, Oxford OX2 9JJ

Printed in the United States of America
British Library Cataloging in Publication Information Available

Library of Congress Cataloging-in-Publication Data

Gennaro, Rocco J.
A dialogue on ethical issues of life and death /
Rocco J. Gennaro.
p. cm
Includes bibliographical references.
1. Life and death, Power over. I. Title.

BJ1469 .G46 2002
179.7—dc21 2002020136 CIP

ISBN 0-7618-2237-2 (pbk. : alk. paper)

The paper used in this publication meets the minimum requirements of American National Standard for Information Sciences—Permanence of Paper for Printed Library Materials, ANSI Z39.48—1984

Dedicated to the memory of my mother, Marian Astuti Gennaro, who gave me life and so much more.

CONTENTS

PREFACE

The way that human beings *ought* to behave is the subject matter of ethics. No inquiry could be more important for intelligent, rational, and civilized beings. This dialogue is an introduction to ethical theory and to four major moral issues: euthanasia, abortion, animal rights, and capital punishment. It is primarily intended for use in ethics and philosophy courses at all levels, but can also be used in law or political science courses. Its main purpose is to develop some of the views and arguments that have emerged in the literature, although I do sometimes present further problems and issues that I have not yet encountered in published work. For those not familiar with the formal discussion on these ethical problems, the dialogue aims to provide an overview of the key issues and is, hopefully, a thought provoking and entertaining work. No prior knowledge of philosophy is required. For those with a broader background, it can serve as a summary of the issues or as a teaching tool.

There are four characters: Larry, Maria, Mark, and Carol. The names were chosen partly so that the reader can more easily remember the basic point of view of each participant by the first letter of his or her name. Thus, *L*arry is rather *l*iberal, and is not very religious. On the other hand, *C*arol is a religious *c*onservative. *M*aria and *M*ark tend to be more *m*oderate in their views, although Maria is moderate to liberal and a believer in God whereas Mark is a moderate conservative and an atheist. The spectrum of opinion is especially clear with respect to the euthanasia and abortion topics. Concerning animals, Maria is the primary advocate for animal rights and vegetarianism. On capital punishment, Carol and Larry are opposed to it whereas Maria and Mark favor the death penalty for certain crimes.

Obviously, I tried to avoid stereotypes, e.g. "all Christians are pro-life," "liberals are soft on crime," and so on. On the other hand, the characters must hold some position, but the reader should not take their positions as ones which all those of their "type" believe. The same goes for their professions. For example, Larry is a lawyer and Carol is a doctor. Clearly, we should not take them as representing their entire professions: there are liberal doctors and conservative lawyers. The reason for choosing their professions mainly has to do with relevant areas of expertise on the issues that arise in the dialogue.

It is unlikely, though certainly possible, that very many readers will agree with one of the characters on everything throughout the entire dialogue. However, my hope is that readers will gain a sense of which position they believe is most defensible on each issue, and one may eventually find oneself tending to agree with one of the characters most of the time. For that reason, I have attempted to keep the conversations continuous in the sense that the same four characters appear throughout the book and they are sometimes reminded of what they have said on the other issues. As we all know, consistency in one's viewpoint is important and we often struggle with questions such as "Can a pro-lifer on abortion be in favor of capital punishment?" or "Can an animal rights activist be pro-choice on abortion?"

The reader should also not be of the impression that the four positions are exhaustive on each issue. There may sometimes be another, or fifth, position that one finds preferable to the four presented. However, it seemed to me that four characters were enough to convey the major views on these topics without oversimplifying or over complicating the issues. Also, although the debate occurs in the United States and most legal references are to our laws and the Constitution, there is some mention of foreign countries when it is particularly appropriate.

Key terms or principles are printed in **bold**; other emphasized words are in *italics*. There is also a Bibliographical Essay at the end of the book, which is where some of the real participants in the dialogue are identified. To keep this book at a manageable length, I obviously had to end the debate at points where others may have continued. However, whenever possible, I pushed the issue as far as I thought was important given the current literature. Indeed, in some places, my hope is that the characters pursued matters in ways that go beyond the reader's initial expectations. Of course, part of the overall purpose is to stimulate debate on these central issues while forcing each of us to examine our own ethical beliefs and presuppositions.

I would like to thank Neil Manson, Donna Franklin, Joe Grcic, and Deborah Wilkes for comments on a previous draft of this manuscript. Special thanks to Judy Barad and Paul Sauer for extensive comments on an earlier draft as well as for many helpful conversations on these ethical issues. Thanks also to Donna Dunbar for her help in the preparation of the camera-ready manuscript.

THE SETTING

Our four characters (Larry, Maria, Mark, and Carol) meet at an International Conference on Ethics and the Law at the Marriott Marquis Hotel in New York City. They had not seen each other for many years, but were good friends while attending college together years earlier in New York City. Larry is now a defense attorney with a New York City law firm after spending several years as a prosecutor. Maria is a professor of psychology at a Pennsylvania University. Mark is a paleontologist and lives in Wyoming, though he frequently travels around the world. Carol is a pediatrician with a private practice in Florida.

THE FIRST DAY

ETHICAL THEORIES

The scene is the registration area at the hotel. Carol is registering for the conference as Larry is walking by the tables.

1. Introduction

LARRY: Carol, is that you?

CAROL: Yes. Hello Larry. How have you been? It's been a while.

LARRY: I'm doing fine. It's been at least seven or eight years. What are you doing here?

CAROL: I'm participating in a panel discussion on abortion.

LARRY: I'm presenting a paper on some legal problems with capital punishment. It's not until the fifth day of the conference, but I wanted to come early and go to other papers and events.

CAROL: I don't participate until the day after tomorrow, but I'm also very interested in other issues, such as euthanasia.

LARRY: Let's get together this evening in the hotel bar. I'm meeting Mark and Maria there at about eight o'clock.

CAROL: Really? They're here too?

LARRY: Yes. I saw them at the book exhibit earlier. Mark is visiting friends and relatives for a few weeks and couldn't resist spending some time here. He has some interest in environmental ethics and abortion. And Mary is presenting a paper on animal rights and consciousness.

CAROL: That sounds great. I haven't looked too closely at the detailed conference program. Anyway, I'll see you there tonight. We'll catch up on old times and perhaps discuss ethics.

LARRY: You can count on that. See you later.

CAROL: Yes.

The scene is the hotel bar at eight o'clock. Larry and Carol are already seated at a table near the bar after having ordered some drinks. Mark and Maria enter the bar together.

MARK: Hello again, Larry. And Carol -- what are you doing here?

CAROL: I'm involved in an abortion panel discussion. It was a good excuse to come up from Florida and visit the Big Apple again.

MARK: I know what you mean after spending so much time in Wyoming and other places around the world.

CAROL: And how are you, Maria?

MARIA: Good. I'm really looking forward to the conference. I love the book exhibits and the whole atmosphere. As an unexpected bonus, I'll be able to spend some time with old friends.

LARRY: Yes, this is nice. We really should have tried to keep in touch more over the past few years, but it's often difficult.

MARIA: Well, let's at least try to make the most of this week together.

MARK: Right. By the way, I hope all of you did a little preparation. I looked over some of my old ethics books as well as some current material.

LARRY: Some of these issues are related to legal matters. That aspect interests me.

MARIA: I'm curious to find out what you now think about some of these controversial issues. We really haven't discussed them in a long time. I'm disturbed, for example, with the way that humans treat other animals. I don't eat meat and I really object to animal experimentation.

CAROL: Abortion is a big issue for me.

MARK: How about we start tonight by getting clear on basic terminology and then we can go over some ethical theories?

LARRY: Fine, and then we can meet every night to discuss a different issue.

CAROL: Sure.

The drinks arrive for Larry and Carol along with a bowl of chips and pretzels. Mark and Maria order their drinks.

MARIA: Maybe we should first just define what ethics is concerned with; namely, the way that human beings *ought* to behave.

MARK: How we *should* behave is not always the same as the way we *actually* behave. People shouldn't murder other people, but murders actually occur all the time.

LARRY: Ethics is concerned with the way that we ought to act even if we don't always live up to it.

CAROL: And when someone doesn't act ethically, then that person is usually said to be doing something morally wrong. On the other hand, a person who does act ethically is doing something right.

MARIA: Sure, but we should also distinguish between what is ethical and what is legal. Larry, you mentioned earlier that ethics is related to the law.

LARRY: That's right. What our society believes to be wrong is reflected in the law and public policy. Rape is against the law because we believe it's wrong. That is a case where what is unethical is illegal.

MARIA: Okay, but my point for now is that what is ethical or moral is not necessarily legal and what is unethical or immoral is not necessarily illegal.

CAROL: True, slavery was legal in this country for years but it was still wrong or unethical. I'd say the same about abortion now.

MARIA: I'd say that about animal experimentation.

LARRY: I'd say that about capital punishment.

MARK: I guess the point is that we each sometimes believe that a law isn't right and should be changed.

MARIA: It goes in the other direction too: there are some illegal behaviors that many people would like to see legalized. For example, physician assisted suicide is illegal in the United States, but many of us don't think it should be. I don't believe it's wrong for a doctor to help a patient die under certain conditions.

LARRY: Let's not forget that the law can often be very helpful in spelling out why a society thinks that something is right or wrong. For example, there are judicial rulings detailing the reasons for the laws that we have. They often contain insightful ethical and philosophical reasoning supporting a particular position.

MARK: I guess a good example could be some of the opinions handed down by the Supreme Court.

LARRY: Exactly. And there has always been a close relation between the concept of justice and the concept of what is right or good.

CAROL: I agree, but we still have to remember that the Supreme Court's primary job is to determine what is constitutional according to our Constitution. This often involves a significant degree of interpretation, and, as we saw with the slavery example, sometimes the Constitution itself needs to be amended.

MARIA: Yes. If a country had a Constitution that said it was fine to rape and assault women, then raping women would be legal in that country. However, whether or not raping women is morally right is another matter entirely.

The drinks arrive for Mark and Maria.

2. Ethical Egoism

MARK: Anyway, let's discuss some ethical theories; that is, answers to the questions "What makes an action right?" and "What makes an action wrong?"

LARRY: That's a good way to put it. Even when we all agree that something is wrong, such as murder or rape, we still need to answer the more fundamental question of *why* it is wrong.

CAROL: And even when we all agree that something is right, such as feeding one's children or keeping one's promises, we still should be able to explain why we think it's right.

MARIA: Let's assume for now that there are absolute and objective moral truths. That is, if an action is right, then it is right for all people everywhere and at all times. And if an action is morally wrong, then it is wrong everywhere and at all times. Let's call this **ethical absolutism**. The idea is that all people are accountable to certain objective and universal moral standards.

LARRY: Okay, but I'd like to discuss relativism later today.

MARIA: Sure, but even among ethical absolutists, there have been various answers to our questions, Mark. Even when we agree that something is wrong, we may disagree about what makes it wrong. And that's why we end up with different ethical theories in the history of philosophy.

MARK: I first wanted to mention a view called **ethical egoism**. It says that "it is morally right for a person to do act X if and only if X has good consequences for that person." And so X would be wrong if X doesn't have good consequences for that person. For example, I should keep my promises because that will have good consequences for me: people will trust me, I will have more friends, etc.

LARRY: Are you an ethical egoist, Mark?

MARK: No, but I don't think it gets the attention it deserves in the literature that I've read. It's often attacked unfairly.

CAROL: Why? Because ethical egoism sounds like a very selfish view of ethical behavior?

MARK: I can understand why it seems that way. After all, the theory basically says that you should do what is in your own self-interest. So it seems to hold that we should all "look out for number one" and care only for how our actions affect ourselves.

MARIA: Egoism does sound that way to me. And it clashes with what I'd consider to be an important aspect of any ethical theory: impartiality. A good ethical theory shouldn't favor any group or individual over others; it should apply equally to everyone.

MARK: That's exactly what prevents me from being an egoist. What makes an act of mine right or wrong should not only depend on how it affects me, but also on how it affects everyone.

LARRY: Then why did you say that egoism gets unfairly attacked?

MARK: Because it seems to me that treating others well is ultimately in one's own self-interest. If murdering my neighbor is wrong, the egoist can agree because killing my neighbor will lead to bad consequences for me. So the egoist need not be selfish at all and should treat others as well as anyone else does. We should distinguish selfish behavior from acting in one's own self-interest. I'm not so sure acting out of self-interest is so terrible; as a matter of fact, we often think that way.

CAROL: But now you are making a psychological claim; namely, that people, as a matter of psychological fact, act out of what they think is in their self-interest. Let's call this **psychological egoism**.

MARK: So? What's the problem?

CAROL: Well, first of all, even if psychological egoism is true, it is no longer an ethical position. Remember that we're concerned with how people ought to behave and not merely with how we actually think or behave.

MARK: Of course.

CAROL: Second, I don't think that psychological egoism is true, especially if it is taken as making a strong universal claim about all human beings.

MARIA: I agree, Carol. I find it hard to believe that all or even most people are always actually thinking about their own self-interest when they make moral decisions. I don't think that way when I do something for my kids. I doubt Mother Teresa walks around thinking "what's in it for me".

MARK: But aren't you and Mother Teresa still doing something that is in your self-interest? If you didn't take care of your kids properly, then you would suffer in the end. Wouldn't you?

MARIA: But that's not *why* I do it. My motivation in doing things for my kids is not one of self-interest. And I'm sure Mother Teresa isn't motivated by self-interest.

MARK: I'm not so sure that there isn't some self-interested motivation; for example, "if I do this, then it will make me feel good." People do get pleasure out of doing things for others, not to mention the fact that it might help you get into Heaven if you are a believer in such things.

CAROL: I believe in Heaven.

MARIA: Me too.

CAROL: But I agree with Maria that even if you're right, Mark, I don't think one's motivation to do good things for others is always self-interest.

MARK: Maybe you're right that it's not always one's conscious motive, but the fact remains that people do get pleasure out of doing things for others and will often feel badly if they don't. But I'm willing to drop it here.

3. Utilitarianism

LARRY: Good. Let's move on to utilitarianism. It's probably the best known ethical theory that also takes the consequences of an action to be crucial. You know, John Stuart Mill and Jeremy Bentham?

MARIA: But there are two different kinds: act-utilitarianism and rule-utilitarianism. Right?

LARRY: Yes, first let's get clear about the general idea which has always been very influential in the way we think about ethical issues.

CAROL: The main idea is that "it is morally right for a person to do act X if and only if X produces more good than bad for everyone affected by the act, including that person." Otherwise, the act would be wrong.

LARRY: That's the basic idea behind **act-utilitarianism**. That is, a person ought to do the act which will bring about a greater balance of good over bad. For example, a person shouldn't rape a woman because the suffering it will cause to the woman and her loved ones will far outweigh any twisted pleasure gained on the part of the rapist.

MARK: And the utilitarian wants us to consider all of the consequences of the action, including long term ones.

LARRY: Right. They are not just concerned with the short term pleasure or good.

MARIA: We should be clear about the terms 'good' and 'bad'.

CAROL: For our purposes, I think it's good enough to think of "good" as meaning 'happiness' or 'pleasure' and "bad" as meaning 'suffering' or 'pain'. That's the way most utilitarians think of it.

LARRY: It's a system of pluses and minuses. When I'm trying to decide whether I'm doing something right or wrong, I should think about the balance of pleasure and pain that will follow from the act. If the pleasure outweighs the pain, the action is right. If not, it's wrong.

CAROL: But there are two major problems with act-utilitarianism. *First*, I don't see how we could know all of the consequences every time that we make an ethical decision. It's a serious practical problem. It would be better if we could just follow certain moral rules or principles.

LARRY: You're right that we can't possibly know all the consequences of an action, but we do the best we can. Sometimes we can rely on history; for example, we know the misery that slavery caused.

CAROL: Of course we often think like utilitarians, but we shouldn't consider *only* the consequences of our actions when we think about what's right or wrong.

MARIA: Let's also not forget that there is an important complication in calculating what we ought to do.

LARRY: What's that?

MARIA: Mill says that there are many different kinds of pleasures and some are "higher" than others.

LARRY: That's right, there are mental and bodily pleasures. There is the pleasure of listening to Beethoven or appreciating fine art as opposed to the pleasure of eating a sandwich. They're both pleasures, but listening to Beethoven is a higher pleasure. Utilitarians don't talk only about immediate or momentary bodily pleasures.

MARIA: Right. It's not only the *quantity* of pleasures that counts but also the *quality* or kind of pleasure. Other factors would include the duration and the intensity of pleasures. But utilitarians do have a difficult time incorporating the quality of pleasures into their quantitative "weighing pluses and minuses" approach.

MARK: But if we need to know which pleasure is higher, we can just find someone who has experienced both pleasures and ask her which is preferable. Just don't ask anyone too young. Most young people prefer bodily pleasures: they have yet to compare them to the so-called "finer things in life."

LARRY: And it's those higher mental pleasures that separate us from other animals. A pig can't appreciate fine art but can get pleasure out of sex and food. That's why Mill went so far as to say "it is better to be a human being dissatisfied than a pig satisfied."

MARIA: And "it is better to be Socrates dissatisfied than a fool satisfied."

LARRY: Right.

MARK: What really differentiates utilitarianism from egoism is that utilitarianism requires us to take into account the happiness or pleasure of *all* those affected by our action, not merely our own happiness.

LARRY: Yes, we need to keep that in mind.

CAROL: But there is a *second* more serious objection to act-utilitarianism.

LARRY: What?

CAROL: It's a theory that can lead to bizarre cases where one's fundamental rights can be violated by an action that act-utilitarians would have to say is right.

MARIA: Like what?

CAROL: Suppose that ten men decide to beat a homeless man to death. They get a certain degree of twisted pleasure out of it. Suppose the suffering of the homeless man is equal to the happiness of one of the men. Suppose too that no one else will really suffer over the loss of the homeless man, since he has no family.

LARRY: What's the point?

CAROL: An act-utilitarian would have to say that such a horrible act is right because it will bring about more pleasure than suffering. But that's absurd. The act would be a violation of the man's right to life. We could easily imagine similar cases that would reduce act-utilitarianism to absurdity.

LARRY: I suppose so, but what if these men were caught and thrown in jail? Then their suffering would probably outweigh the pleasure experienced from the act.

CAROL: Sure, but it's a poor theory that says this act is wrong only if the men are caught and thrown in jail. What they did was wrong, period!

MARIA: Here's another case: we could imagine a situation where one business man A kills a business enemy B. B has no family and few friends whereas A has a wife and several kids. A's killing B leads to tremendous prosperity for A, which is passed down to his children and their children and so on. Again, it would seem that, as long as A is not caught, A actually did something right according to the act-utilitarian. That does seem absurd.

LARRY: That it does.

CAROL: The general problem seems to be focusing exclusively on good and bad consequences. That can lead to individual cases where violating a basic right is the right thing to do, or at least it's not automatically wrong.

MARK: Wouldn't it be better to focus on the consequences of following the general *principle* "do not murder"?

MARIA: Yes; that's closer to what's called **rule-utilitarianism,** which says that we should act in accordance with rules that tend to increase happiness and diminish suffering. For example, we should follow the rule "do not kill your business rivals" which, generally, will lead to greater happiness or reduced suffering even if the opposite would happen in a particular case. This is the way rule-utilitarianism avoids the major problem with act-utilitarianism.

MARK: I think rule-utilitarianism also reflects more accurately the important connection between ethics and the law that Larry spoke of earlier. We can think of many of our laws as rules which, if followed, would tend to increase happiness and diminish suffering.

LARRY: Exactly. And I think people use this reasoning frequently when debating a law. For example, people debate the legalization of certain drugs. Rule-utilitarianism would tell us to think about the consequences of following such a rule as "legalize marijuana and cocaine." Of course, utilitarians may disagree among themselves about whether or not such a law would really lessen suffering rather than increase it, but that's often how the debate goes.

CAROL: I agree that rule-utilitarianism is superior to act-utilitarianism, but it can suffer from the same sort of weakness. It might justify rules that are unjust. For example, if all businesses adopted the rule "only promote white males and females, not blacks or Hispanics" a rule-utilitarian might be forced to admit that this would generally lead to more happiness over suffering simply because the large majority of the worker population is white. Their happiness will outweigh the suffering of minorities.

MARK: I see the problem. It's similar to the main problem with act-utilitarianism, although in this case individual rights can be trampled on in the name of a general principle.

CAROL: Right.

MARIA: And sometimes it's difficult to know how to formulate the rule. If it's too general, it won't be flexible enough to tell us what to do in particular cases. If it's too specific, it won't apply in any other circumstance. There is the danger that rule-utilitarianism will simply collapse into act-utilitarianism if the rules become specific enough to handle exceptional circumstances. Nonetheless, I still think that rule-utilitarianism is probably closest to the truth.

More drinks and snacks are ordered, and they arrive within a few minutes.

4. Kant's Theory

MARK: Despite my attempt to defend egoism, I'm most sympathetic to Immanuel Kant's theory.

LARRY: Which one?

MARK: The **Categorical Imperative**. It says that an act is morally right if and only if the maxim of the act can be willed to become a universal law of nature. Categorical imperatives are *unconditional*, such as "keep your promises" or "do not lie"; they don't depend on conditions or circumstances. The only unconditional good is a *good will* from which all rational beings should act. Other goods, such as intelligence and perseverance, can be used for bad purposes. But the good will is, for Kant, one that's directed toward doing one's duty. The categorical imperative is the basic principle that enables us to determine what our duty is.

CAROL: Yes, he gives several examples to illustrate how to formulate and follow a Categorical Imperative in a particular case. I like the one he uses to show that suicide is wrong. How does it go?

MARK: The maxim or rule "from self-love I wish to shorten my life because it is likely to bring about more evil than satisfaction" cannot be willed to be a universal law of nature. It would be contradictory.

CAROL: Right. Kant is asking "What if everyone lived by that rule or maxim?" Often the result would either be disastrous or contradictory in some sense. Obviously, everyone could not "live" by that maxim.

LARRY: Interesting.

MARIA: Doesn't he give another example about someone who promises to repay borrowed money knowing that he would not repay it?

MARK: Yes. Kant again shows how acting in accordance with such a maxim would ultimately contradict itself.

LARRY: How's that?

MARK: Well, what would happen to the whole concept or idea of promising if everyone behaved in such a way?

LARRY: I guess it would crumble because ultimately no one would take anyone's promise seriously.

MARK: Exactly, and so Kant says that we should "keep our promises" unconditionally and without regard to particular circumstances.

LARRY: That sounds good, but his theory suffers from some of the same problems that weaken rule-utilitarianism. How do we formulate these rules or maxims in a way that's not too general and not too specific?

MARK: I think Kant would make them very general in the way that we've already seen.

LARRY: But then his position is a bit extreme. Is it *always* wrong to kill oneself? Is it *always* wrong to lie, say, even to save someone's life?

MARK: Good questions. Kant would answer yes to both of them. I share your discomfort, but I think it's far better than the other ethical theories we've discussed so far. I agree, though, that Kant did not seem to consider what to do when we have *conflicting* duties, such as saving a life and keeping a promise.

MARIA: I'm confused. It sounds like Kant's theory is very close to rule-utilitarianism. The Categorical Imperative tells us to act in accordance with rules or maxims that lead to the best consequences, and to avoid those actions, such as lying, which would lead to bad consequences if everyone followed them. Isn't Kant relying too heavily on consequences?

MARK: I suppose so, but there is another very important aspect to Kant's theory which really distinguishes it from any form of utilitarianism.

MARIA: What's that?

MARK: For various reasons Kant believed that the Categorical Imperative presupposed the absolute worth of rational beings. He makes it clear that we should treat people as *ends* in themselves and not as mere *means* to promote an end. It is disrespectful to treat people as a means to one's ends. Basically, "using people" for one's own benefit is wrong.

CAROL: So, for Kant, killing the business rival or homeless person we spoke of earlier is wrong partly because killing someone is treating them as a means to an end.

MARK: It's not merely the consequences of "pleasure" and "suffering" that make an act right or wrong. It's most importantly the fact that we treat each other as intrinsically valuable beings. In that way, Kant can better account for those important individual rights that cause so many problems for utilitarianism.

CAROL: Yes, we shouldn't have to think first about the consequences of a man raping a woman or burning down her house to know that such actions are wrong. They are unjust and immoral actions, Kant would say, because of the disrespectful manner in which the man has treated the woman as a means to his end.

MARK: Exactly.

5. God's Command

CAROL: If it weren't for my belief in God, then perhaps I'd also be most sympathetic to Kant's theory, but I think that morality must be more closely tied to God and religion.

LARRY: How so? You know I'm not very religious, although I do have great interest in various Eastern religions and philosophy. I don't believe in a conscious all-powerful creator God.

MARK: Neither do I. I'd have to say that I'm an atheist for reasons that we can discuss some other time.

MARIA: I believe in God, but I'm not sure that I will agree with Carol about the relation between religion and morality.

LARRY: Well, what did you have in mind, Carol?

CAROL: It seems to me that what is right or wrong has to be ultimately grounded in a belief in an all-good and all-knowing God. God determines what is wrong and what is right. We then ought to follow God's commands.

LARRY: Are you saying, for example, that what makes murder wrong is the fact that God says that it's wrong?

CAROL: Yes. Let's call it the **God's Command** theory of ethics: An act is wrong because God says that it's wrong; and an act is right because God says that it's right. So, for example, we ought to behave in accordance with the Ten Commandments and Biblical teaching because they are the words and commands of God.

MARK: Well, there are many serious problems with that view, Carol. First of all, you must realize that many people do not share your belief in God. So to base morality entirely on religion and a belief in God will often not be very convincing as a practical matter.

LARRY: Right. And in a country such as ours where there are so many different religious beliefs, your theory is easy to refute under the heading of "freedom of religion."

CAROL: How do you mean?

LARRY: Well, take abortion for example. If you say that the *only* reason why abortion is wrong is the fact that God and your religion says it's wrong, then a person of a different religion can simply reply that her religion does not share such a view.

CAROL: So? I believe that my religion is the correct one.

LARRY: But it would be like trying to convince everyone that contraception is morally wrong based on religion. No such argument would have the practical effect you want it to have. Even worse, if you want to change laws to reflect religious beliefs, you will soon realize that we can't base our laws solely on the views of any one religion. What if a person of another religion argued the same way you do?

CAROL: I see what you mean, but I still think that without a belief in God there would be little reason for many people to act morally.

MARK: Are you saying that atheists can't act morally?

CAROL: No, but some atheists use their lack of belief in God and immortality to "justify" all kinds of immoral activity. Look at Hitler's Germany. I mean, if there is no ultimate punishment or reward in an afterlife, how can anything be truly right or wrong? What would be the point?

MARK: First of all, I can give you just as many examples of people doing horrible things, like burning widows alive and human sacrifice, in the "name of God." Look at the "holy wars." As far as I can see, there is little evidence to suggest that a belief in God or a Supreme Being prompts people to act morally.

CAROL: I'm not so sure about that. There have been many more "unholy" wars than "holy" wars. And don't forget that religious people also do a lot of good in the world.

MARK: Sure but, second, you seem to be making a rather puzzling claim about the source of morality. It sounds like you are making the *psychological* claim that many people *need to believe* in God and immortality in order to behave morally. But fear of punishment, hope of reward, or even love of God don't seem to be the right motives for morality, if you ask me.

LARRY: I agree. It's wrong to steal and kill because they are bad things to do to the victims, not because the consequences for the perpetrator can be unpleasant. Now you sound like the egoist, Carol.

CAROL: I wouldn't say that those are the *only* motives for behaving morally, but I think they're important to many people.

MARK: Anyone who has to believe in God or immortality in order to keep from murdering or raping another person is a psychologically weak person. Maybe there are some people like that, but it's a scary thought. I can't imagine a good religious person thinking "if I stopped believing in God, it would be morally right for me to go out and rape someone."

CAROL: I agree that they shouldn't, but some people would think that way.

MARK: That's pretty disturbing.

LARRY: But the main objection to God's Command theory, going back to Plato, is that God's attitude toward murder or rape is not what *makes* them wrong. Something is not wrong because God forbids it or doesn't like it, but rather God forbids or doesn't like something because it is wrong. Murder is wrong for all sorts of independent reasons, and that's why God forbids it. But God's attitude toward murder is not what makes it wrong.

MARK: Exactly! And, again, what if there is no God? Does it follow that nothing would be right or wrong? Of course not. Is rape suddenly morally permissible? I don't think so. Anyway, there are many non-believers, including myself, who can make perfectly legitimate judgments of right and wrong.

CAROL: You make some good points, but religion is often closely linked to how one thinks one ought to behave.

LARRY: True, religion and morality are often closely associated in people's minds, but to say that morality has to be grounded in religion is quite different.

MARK: Yes. It's true that through one's religious upbringing a person will associate various ethical or non-ethical behaviors with that religion. But it's quite different to say that morality *requires* religion.

CAROL: I'm not so sure, but I'm willing to drop it here. What do you think, Maria? You've been rather quiet. I know you believe in God.

MARIA: I've been intrigued by the conversation. I'd say that belief in God or immortality and God's attitude toward an action is not *the* reason why the action is right or wrong. However, I think God's attitude can be offered as one reason among others. In other words, it's perfectly fine to offer religious reasons against murder without thinking that it's the only, or even the primary, reason murder is wrong.

LARRY: Sure, but then it becomes a reason based more on one's personal or individual faith. It's often difficult to use that reason in order to convince those who don't share one's faith.

MARK: That was your earlier point, right?

LARRY: Yes.

MARIA: The other problem I see with basing morality on religion is simply the fact that many people within a particular religion often disagree very strongly on a given issue. For example, there are pro-choice Christians even though we are usually portrayed as necessarily pro-life in the way that I'm sure Carol prefers.

CAROL: That's right. I would say that being pro-choice is inconsistent with fundamental Christian principles, despite what you might believe.

LARRY: Can we stay on track here?

MARIA: Okay. My main point is that it's difficult to base morality on religion because there tends to be disagreement about what the true religious doctrines are.

CAROL: But surely there are certain fundamental beliefs in every religion, aren't there? If one doesn't share them, then one is free to find another. Anyway, I don't see how disagreement about whether or not abortion is morally wrong means that morality shouldn't be based on religion? I mean, all utilitarians don't agree on these issues either, but we didn't treat that as an objection.

MARIA: Good point, but religion does seem different. Rule-utilitarians may disagree about whether or not capital punishment is wrong because they may have calculated its consequences differently, but here we are disagreeing about the religious doctrine itself.

MARK: I agree with Maria. The way I would put it is that God's Command theory faces the additional practical problem of knowing exactly what God's attitudes are in certain cases. As Maria said, even within a religion there can be significant disagreement between so-called "expert" Biblical scholars.

CAROL: Well, I'll listen to what the Pope has to say. That's a good starting point for me. Not all Biblical interpretations are equally valid.

MARIA: You know, sometimes I wonder if the whole "action-based" approach is wrong.

LARRY: How so?

MARIA: Why not follow the **virtue ethics** model and ask "What kind of person should I be?" instead of "What should I do?"

CAROL: So we should strive to acquire the virtues, such as compassion and honesty, and we would all be happier in the end.

LARRY: Well, being a virtuous person is certainly a noble goal, but I think we still need an ethical theory that tells us what we ought *to do* on particular occasions. So I am not sure we can really separate virtue ethics and action-based theories.

MARK: I agree. Being an honest person is great, but the action-based point remains: Follow the rule "do not lie" in particular circumstances.

MARIA: I suppose so, but there is much more to virtue ethics than that.

6. Relativism

LARRY: Sure, but so far we have assumed that if an action is right it is *objectively* right for all people everywhere and at all times. And if an action is morally wrong, it's objectively wrong everywhere and at all times. We called this "ethical absolutism." The idea is that all people are accountable to certain universal moral standards, even if people disagree about what they are.

CAROL: I'm certainly an ethical absolutist. Aren't you?

MARK: Yes.

MARIA: Yes.

LARRY: I guess I'm a bit unsure. I find relativism more attractive than you do.

MARK: How do you understand ethical relativism?

LARRY: **Ethical relativism** says that morality is culturally defined. More specifically, an act is right in some culture or group C if and only if it is normal or generally accepted in C. Whether or not an action is right depends upon where and when it occurs; that is, it depends on whether or not it is accepted in that culture at that time.

MARIA: Like what?

LARRY: Polygamy is normal or accepted in some countries, but not in the United States. So polygamy would be wrong here, but not in those countries where it's accepted. You find a similar situation throughout the world with homosexuality. Even such behaviors as headhunting and human sacrifice are or have been accepted in certain cultures. Morality is just a term for socially approved or accepted customs, and so morality too is culturally defined. Moral standards vary from culture to culture and from time to time. Morality is relative to time and place. There is no absolute right or wrong.

MARIA: It's true that different cultures have different beliefs and customs, but that is merely a sociological fact. It sounds like a confusion of law and ethics. I really don't see how ethical relativism can stand up to criticism.

LARRY: Try me.

MARIA: In some cases it leads to absurd consequences. There are well-known objections to it that take the form of a **reductio ad absurdum** argument. The idea is to assume that some theory is true for the sake of argument, then show that it leads to an absurd conclusion. We should then conclude that the theory is false. It's a common form of argument.

LARRY: Yes, but can you give an example in the case of ethical relativism?

MARIA: Sure, but first, I assume that when you say "what is generally accepted in a culture" you mean "what the majority in that culture believe to be right."

LARRY: Yes, the relativist is saying that what most people think is right in a culture C at a time t is what is right in C at t. And what most people think is wrong in C at t is wrong.

MARIA: But that leads to the conclusion that the majority in a culture can never be wrong. That's absurd. I mean, can't the majority ever be mistaken?

LARRY: I see the problem.

MARIA: If ethical relativism is correct, then it would be impossible for the majority of moral beliefs of a society to be wrong. So if a culture believed that raping women was right, then it would be right to do in that culture? I can't accept that.

CAROL: And if the majority is always right, then any moral reformer, such as Jesus or Martin Luther King, would automatically be wrong and acting immorally. That is also absurd.

LARRY: But most people did think they were wrong at the time.

MARIA: Perhaps, but the problem for relativism is that it equates what *is right or wrong* with what some people *think is right or wrong*. What is right can't be discovered merely by an opinion poll at a particular time. The majority might be right, but they also might not be. The relativist can't make that important distinction. According to relativism, if most people think rape is right in country A, then it is right in country A. If most people think that rape is wrong in country B, then it is wrong in country B. Sounds like nonsense to me.

MARK: Me too. Rape is simultaneously right in country A, but wrong in country B. That can't be correct. If you said that most people *believe or think* that rape is right in A and wrong in B, that's fine. But it's very different to say that rape *is* right in A and wrong in B.

CAROL: The relativist's line of argument is invalid anyway. From the fact that two cultures believe differently about what is right, it doesn't follow that there is no objective truth of the matter. That's a terrible form of argument. Consider this: culture A believes that 20 + 20 = 40 but culture B believes that 20 + 20 = 42; therefore, 20 + 20 = 40 in culture A, but it equals 42 in culture B. Or: culture A believes that the Earth is round, but culture B believes that it's flat; therefore, the Earth is round in culture A but flat in culture B. Ridiculous!

LARRY: Maybe, but I'm not sure that ethical "truths" deserve to be placed on a par with mathematical or scientific truths. Your examples use clearly objective facts where one culture is obviously wrong, but where is the similarity to ethics here?

CAROL: The logical point is the same. Just because there are different beliefs, it doesn't follow that there is no objective truth about the issue at hand.

MARK: Right. I think relativists confuse the claim that it is often difficult *to know* what is right or wrong with the claim that *there are* no absolute moral truths. The former is true since we do often argue and disagree about ethical issues, but the latter is false and clearly doesn't follow from the former.

LARRY: You could be right. Maybe it's just that there is so much disagreement about ethical issues that I start to wonder "Is there really an objective answer to some of these questions?"

MARIA: Well, that brings me to another absurd consequence of relativism. The fact that we disagree about ethical issues actually supports ethical absolutism, not relativism.

LARRY: How?

MARIA: If we really thought that there were no objective ethical truths, then no genuine moral disagreements or comparisons would be possible. I mean, how could we truly disagree about, say, the ethics of abortion, if there were no objective truth? To put it another way: how could two cultures really be *disagreeing* over abortion if what is right or wrong is purely culturally defined?

CAROL: Right, if relativism were true, then ethical differences would be more like differences in food tastes among different cultures. But clearly when we disagree over human rights, abortion, capital punishment, and so on, we aren't merely saying something analogous to "one culture likes to eat snakes but another culture does not." Ethical disagreement goes deeper and clearly presupposes objective truth, even if it's difficult to discover.

LARRY: I see, but I'm still not sure that it's the same as mathematical or scientific disagreement.

MARK: Also, if relativism were true we couldn't criticize the morals of another culture, or *vice versa*. That seems ridiculous. The morality of all cultures would be the same because there is nothing right or wrong as such.

MARIA: Yes. We can still be respectful and understanding of other cultures and their practices or customs without holding that all cultures at all times are morally equal.

CAROL: That reminds me of one more related objection to relativism.

LARRY: What?

CAROL: Well, did most people in the United States believe that slavery was right or morally permissible in, say, the 1830's?

LARRY: I suppose so.

CAROL: What about now?

LARRY: Obviously not. With the possible exception of some lunatic racist groups, slavery is widely believed to be wrong today.

CAROL: So have we progressed morally since slavery days on this issue?

LARRY: Sure.

CAROL: But if you are truly a relativist you can't make that claim.

LARRY: I see. Because in order to acknowledge moral progress, there must be some objective moral standard against which such a judgment can be made.

MARIA: Right. A relativist would have to say that slavery was right in the 1830's and slavery is wrong now. That's it. Unlike the absolutist, the relativist can't say that slavery is wrong, period, regardless of what an ignorant culture may have believed at a particular time.

LARRY: When you put it like that I am very uncomfortable with relativism.

MARK: I guess if you are a relativist, then you really shouldn't argue with us. Just take a poll and that's it. Right?

LARRY: Very funny, but I plan to argue for my positions very strongly.

MARK: I thought so. That proves you really aren't a relativist at heart. After all, you said earlier that you oppose capital punishment while the majority of Americans today apparently favor it. So you obviously believe that the majority can be mistaken, at least sometimes. Right?

LARRY: I guess so.

CAROL: One last point. There is a real problem with the idea of a "group" or a "culture." I mean, what constitutes a culture or group anyway? A country? The state you live in? The clubs or organizations that you belong to? Why shouldn't the Mafia be construed as a group or culture entitled to have their own moral standard? It's crazy.

MARIA: I agree. The danger is that ethical relativism will ultimately lead to an even more radical "individual relativism." Each person decides for him or her self what is right or wrong. And if that is so, then even comparative judgments such as "one person acts better than another" become meaningless. All moral standards vanish.

CAROL: Relativism would therefore be disastrous on practical conduct. If we really believed that one moral standard is as good as any other, then we are likely to conclude that any behavior is morally equal to any other.

LARRY: On that note, I need to go. I want to get up early and hear a paper on euthanasia in the morning. I'll see you tomorrow.

MARK: Sure. Take care, Larry. It was good to see you again.

Larry leaves, but Carol, Mark, and Maria stay for another twenty minutes or so catching up on old times. They all plan on attending a session on euthanasia the next day.

THE SECOND DAY

EUTHANASIA

The scene is the hotel bar at eight o'clock. Mark, Mary, Larry and Carol are sitting near the end of the bar with drinks after having just finished dinner with several other conference participants.

1. Terminology and the Law

LARRY: I really enjoyed the day today. How about you, Mark?

MARK: Yes. I listened to an interesting debate on euthanasia. It was part of a longer session on the topic.

LARRY: I was there too. It was crowded. And then I went to another talk on the current law. I still can't believe that, in a country like ours, active voluntary euthanasia and assisted suicide are illegal.

CAROL: I have the feeling that we are going to disagree, Larry.

MARY: It sounds like I'll be more on Larry's side.

MARK: If we are going to debate the topic, perhaps we should first be clear about some terminology and the current United States law.

MARIA: Of course. Well, there is the distinction between voluntary and nonvoluntary euthanasia. **Voluntary euthanasia** is when euthanasia is performed in response to the informed request of a competent patient. In short, the patient asks for euthanasia. On the other hand, **nonvoluntary euthanasia** is when euthanasia is performed on an individual who does not request death; for example, a mentally incompetent adult suffering from a mental illness or a severely ill infant who is incapable of giving consent.

CAROL: That's an important difference.

LARRY: We should also note the distinction between passive and active euthanasia.

MARK: **Passive euthanasia** is to allow a patient to die; for example, by withholding or withdrawing a respirator. **Active euthanasia** is killing the patient; for example, with the lethal injection of a drug.

LARRY: Theoretically, then, there are four types of euthanasia: voluntary active, nonvoluntary active, voluntary passive, and nonvoluntary passive.

CAROL: But isn't passive euthanasia, whether it's voluntary or nonvoluntary, relatively uncontroversial?

LARRY: Yes, especially voluntary passive. We already have a fairly well established system of so-called "advance directives" such as "living wills." They establish in advance specific instructions about a person's care should life-sustaining treatment ever be needed. Mentally competent adults long have had the right in this country to refuse treatment in certain cases. And there is also a "proxy directive" where a person specifies someone else to make health care decisions for him or her in case the decision-making capacity is lost.

MARIA: Why is nonvoluntary passive euthanasia still somewhat controversial?

LARRY: It may involve withholding life-sustaining treatment from, say, mentally or physically defective newborns. Although I believe that euthanasia in some of these cases is morally justifiable, I can understand why someone might believe that these cases are a bit harder to justify since the patient cannot consent.

MARIA: So is it safe to say that the primary controversy surrounds active euthanasia?

LARRY: Yes, especially active voluntary euthanasia.

CAROL: By the way, let's not forget the American Medical Association position which says that the patient and/or the immediate family can decide whether or not to continue the employment of extraordinary means when there is irrefutable evidence that biological death is imminent. On the other hand, the intentional termination of the life of the patient is against the policy of the AMA and is contrary to that for which the medical profession stands.

MARIA: So the AMA allows for some cases of passive euthanasia, but not for active euthanasia?

CAROL: As far as I know. Active euthanasia is illegal in the United States, whereas passive euthanasia isn't.

2. Killing, Letting Die, and the Relevance of Intentions

LARRY: But I have a real problem with the distinction between passive and active euthanasia.

MARK: In what way?

LARRY: Well, I don't believe that there is a moral difference between "allowing someone to die" and "killing someone," as long as all other circumstances are the same. Suppose that in a case of the imminent death of a bone cancer patient, everyone agrees it is morally permissible to withhold life sustaining measures. What then happens? The patient starves to death or dies of dehydration over a painful period of several days.

CAROL: Usually, yes. Of course, in other cases, such as a coma, no suffering would occur.

LARRY: But if that is morally permissible, then why isn't it also right, once the initial decision has been made to withhold treatment, to actively kill the patient so that he will not unnecessarily suffer for that additional period of time?

CAROL: Because doctors are not supposed to kill their patients.

LARRY: If it's morally permissible to allow them to die, then it should be morally right to kill them under those same conditions. Indeed, it seems cruel to let the bone cancer patient suffer for those extra days when he could be spared the unnecessary suffering. From a utilitarian point of view, euthanasia is clearly right in such cases unless the terminal patient has strong feelings against it. The amount of eliminated suffering outweighs any possible pleasure gained, assuming that there is even any pleasure to be gained at all.

MARK: Are you saying that, generally, there is no moral difference between "letting die" and "killing"?

LARRY: That's right. Think about this: A person, Tom, is behind the wheel of his car intending to run over John who is leaving his apartment late in the evening. John leaves his house and Tom runs him over and kills him. Clearly Tom has done something wrong.

MARK: Of course.

LARRY: Now take another scenario where a different person, Mike, is also behind the wheel of his car intending to run over John. But John leaves his home and accidentally trips down the stairs. John is bleeding to death. Mike goes over to John and simply lets him die without doing anything to help him. Is there any moral difference between the actions or inactions of Tom and Mike? I don't think so. Letting die or killing would, in either case, be wrong.

Similarly, in the case of the bone cancer patient I think that killing him or letting him die are both morally acceptable. My point is that either they are both wrong or they are both right depending on the circumstances. You can't just say that passive euthanasia is morally justifiable and then say that active euthanasia is always wrong.

MARIA: I see, but wouldn't Tom's action be viewed as *more wrong* than what Mike did? At least according to the law, Tom committed first degree murder whereas Mike did not. There are *degrees of wrongness* in the eyes of the law.

LARRY: Yes, but both are still wrong.

CAROL: Sure, but that is one reason why we normally think of killing as worse than letting die, even if we believe various forms of negligence are also wrong.

MARK: I think we are really missing the main point of the AMA policy.

CAROL: How so?

MARK: The key to me is the word 'intentional': the *intentional* termination of life is against the AMA policy. And in your examples, Larry, both Tom and Mike had the intention to kill John. That's what makes both of their actions wrong. The key issue is not the killing/letting die distinction as such, but rather whether or not the termination of life is intentional.

CAROL: So doctors should never intentionally terminate the life of a patient either by direct action or by omission?

MARK: Yes.

LARRY: But why should one's intentions matter in determining whether or not an action is right or wrong? Perhaps we think less of *a person* who has bad intentions, but how is that relevant to whether or not *the action* is right or wrong?

MARIA: We already saw how bad intentions can make a wrong act worse. Also, if I put a drug in your coffee intending to make you sick, that would be wrong. But if I put it in your coffee intending to *kill you*, it would be worse.

LARRY: But how could bad intentions make an otherwise morally permissible act wrong?

MARK: Sometimes we cannot even determine whether an act is right or wrong until we know the intentions of the person. This happens all the time in cases of accidents: if the child accidentally fell out of the window, then the mother probably did not do anything morally wrong. However, if she intentionally threw her child from the window, she did act wrongly.

CAROL: And there are also cases of lying. Perhaps not all instances of lying are wrong, but clearly some are. What makes them wrong? It's mainly that the person is *intentionally* not telling the truth. That's what makes it lying. On the other hand, merely uttering a falsehood without bad intent is not wrong. As Kant might say, we should not treat others as means to our ends, which is usually what happens when one lies.

LARRY: I see, but we must again be careful not to confuse the rightness or wrongness of the act with what we might think of the character of the person.

MARIA: Of course, but it does seem obvious that bad intentioned people are more likely to commit morally wrong acts. People's attitudes, including their intentions, desires and beliefs, will ultimately dictate how they behave towards others.

MARK: That's partly why we don't want doctors to end life intentionally, either actively or passively.

LARRY: But don't doctors intentionally let their patients die all the time? Isn't that how this conversation started?

MARK: Yes. But I don't think the doctor's intention is to end life in the already legal cases of "letting die" or passive euthanasia.

LARRY: Well, they *know* that the patient will die if treatment is withheld. Right?

MARK: Sure, but there is a difference between intentions and knowledge. I'm sure you know this from your legal training.

LARRY: Of course.

MARK: A doctor can *know* that the patient's death will result from withdrawing treatment without *intending* for the patient to die.

MARIA: I like the analogy to driving my car: when I drive my car to work I know that my tires will wear down and that I will use gas, but that is not my intention when I drive to work. My intention is to get to school so that I can teach my classes.

LARRY: Why can't we make the same distinction in a case of *active* euthanasia?

MARIA: Perhaps we can.

LARRY: So a doctor injects the dying patient with a lethal dose without the intention to cause death, but only, say, to relieve suffering. Of course, the doctor knows that she will die, but that is not the doctor's intention. So, again, I see no moral difference between active and passive euthanasia here.

MARIA: Sounds right to me.

CAROL: Not to me. It still seems different to have doctors as *the cause* of the patient's death.

MARK: I agree. In the case of active euthanasia, the fact remains that the doctor and the lethal injection is the cause of the patient's death regardless of how imminent death is. On the other hand, passive euthanasia merely allows the patient to die of the disease or ailment. The disease is the cause of death. That makes a big difference to me.

MARIA: But why?

3. The Sanctity of Life versus the Quality of Life

CAROL: I know Mark will not completely agree with me here, but I believe that it's a matter of *the sanctity of human life*; that is, human life is a sacred gift from God and no one has the right to take it away. Human beings should not be in the business of "playing God" and ending other human lives, no matter what the illness.

MARK: I don't agree with your religious reasons, Carol, but I do agree that human life is intrinsically valuable and should be preserved at virtually all costs. At the least, I don't think that we should begin letting doctors kill patients.

MARIA: I don't agree with you, Carol, even though we share a belief in God. Aren't we already playing God with the use of technology, which allows us to continue lives artificially with respirators and artificial kidneys and hearts?

CAROL: But the difference in those cases is that we are preserving and protecting human life instead of ending it. God wants us to value human life and use our minds to discover cures and medicines.

MARIA: How do you know that God wants us to preserve life at all costs, no matter what the suffering?

CAROL: Maybe I don't, but a strong belief in the sanctity of human life is essential to the Christian faith.

MARIA: I struggle with the idea that God thinks it's right for us to intervene in the health and life of human beings to the point of only prolonged misery, but then God would think it's wrong for us to end that life when death is imminent.

LARRY: I agree with Maria. After all, the patient wouldn't even be in that condition if it weren't for the medical technology in the first place.

CAROL: Sure, but we shouldn't use that as an excuse to kill patients whenever we want.

MARIA: Of course not, but it should be a factor in any ethical decision. What do you think, Mark?

MARK: I see your point, but, of course, I don't think that active euthanasia is wrong for religious reasons. I am just very uncomfortable with the whole idea of licensing doctors to kill their patients. It doesn't seem to be the right kind of thing for doctors to be doing. Their job is to cure and give comfort, not to kill. If someone in pain wants to kill himself, then go ahead, but why involve doctors?

LARRY: Surely, at least sometimes, causing death is the most comforting thing a doctor can do for a patient. Under certain conditions, it might be in the patient's best interest to die.

MARK: Perhaps you're right, but those are relatively rare cases. I guess I don't believe that death is *always* worse than being alive. Also, in cases of apparently irreversible comas, it's really unclear whether or not the patient is "alive" in any important sense. Merely keeping a patient *biologically* alive seems only to prolong the dying process, especially when there is virtually no brain activity. On the other hand, the *person*, in the more important *psychological* sense, has already died as far as I'm concerned.

LARRY: That brings me back to my earlier point. Carol spoke of the "sanctity of life," but what about *the quality of life*? I believe there are some circumstances where the quality of one's life is so poor that it outweighs any so-called 'sanctity' of life.

CAROL: I can't agree.

LARRY: I knew you'd say that. Why must we suppose that a human life should be preserved *no matter what*? If someone is in continuous agony with no chance of recovery, why not let the person die with some dignity? After all, we often associate the term 'euthanasia' with 'mercy killing.' Don't you have any compassion for these people?

CAROL: Of course I do. I see them every day at work. But compassion should not be measured by one's willingness to kill someone. A truly compassionate response to a suffering person's cry for help -- even if that person asks to be killed -- is to do everything possible to cure, comfort, or ease the pain; not to kill the person. That's a deadly form of compassion which is unfortunately used by pro-euthanasia groups to promote their dangerous agenda. They make it sound like you don't care about the suffering of patients unless you are in favor of killing them. What a terrible way to play on people's sympathies and emotions.

LARRY: Oh, come on. That seems unfair.

CAROL: I don't think so. Remember what you just said?

LARRY: Yes, but you know I didn't really mean to accuse you of having no compassion.

CAROL: Maybe.

MARIA: Anyway, let's remember that we're talking about voluntary euthanasia; that is, cases where the patient requests death.

LARRY: Yes. It's not as if we'd be killing patients against their will.

4. Pain and Mental Competence

CAROL: Pain is usually the cause of a desire to die. I'd like to see those who favor euthanasia put as much energy into the area of pain control. As it is, even many doctors are not very well trained in the treatment of pain.

LARRY: That's fine, but not all of the pain from diseases or illnesses can be controlled by medication.

CAROL: As far as I know, most pain can be controlled. But the key issue is the psychological effect severe pain or a severe disability can have on a person; namely, one tends to suffer from episodes of depression. It's somewhat natural to be depressed, especially at first, but should we kill someone who requests death under these conditions? I don't think so.

MARK: I agree with Carol here. We've been speaking of "mentally competent" patients in the context of voluntary euthanasia. But how do we determine whether a patient who is probably depressed is mentally competent enough to make such a request? Who is going to determine the competence of the patient? I have some real problems with these questions.

CAROL: Me too.

LARRY: Why not have a group of psychologists at each hospital? Together with the family of the patient, a decision as to mental competence wouldn't be hard to reach.

MARK: I disagree. It opens another can of worms anyway.

CAROL: You see, Larry, it's all part of the more general problem of rationality. Normally, when someone wants to die, say a teenager ready to jump off a bridge, we think that it's justifiable to intervene because we don't believe that she is thinking rationally. People will say and do all kinds of things when they aren't thinking straight.

MARK: A similar justification can be found in cases where a patient requests death. People do change their minds. You know that well over ninety percent of those who are prevented from committing suicide are later very glad that they were kept from killing themselves.

MARIA: You may be right for a typical attempted suicide, but in those cases the person is not in intolerable physical pain and is not terminally ill. I think that those two conditions must be present in order for active voluntary euthanasia to be carried out.

LARRY: And the problem of mental competence can be dealt with by psychologists, families, and lawyers over a long period of time so that no rash decisions are made. After all, as you know, mental competence hearings occur every day in court cases where a defendant's mental state is in question.

MARK: I think you're too optimistic, but I'm sure that your lawyer and psychologist friends would appreciate the extra work!

CAROL: As it is, doctors often don't know where they stand in the eyes of the law. We are paranoid of law suits. That's why malpractice insurance is so high and why we often run expensive tests when they are probably unnecessary. Bringing in more lawyers will only make it worse.

LARRY: I don't agree. I think it would help to make it clear where one stands.

CAROL: I find that hard to believe. It's fairly simple and clear now: no doctor should kill a patient no matter how much the patient requests it.

They each order another drink and it arrives quickly, although Carol and Larry opt for a non-alcoholic beverage.

5. The Principle of Autonomy versus the Principle of Beneficence

LARRY: Let's approach this issue from a related point of view. You reminded me of it when you spoke of attempted suicide.

CAROL: What's that?

LARRY: As you probably know, there are two important moral principles that are always potentially in conflict. They are also important in legal and political philosophy.

MARIA: What are they?

LARRY: On the one hand, there is the **principle of autonomy** which says that people ought to be able to do what they want provided that their actions don't harm others or themselves. The idea is crucial to our individual liberty and freedom. People ought to be respected as self-determining moral agents. Indeed, the word 'autonomy' comes from the Greek words *autos* meaning "self" and *nomos* meaning "law." So the idea is "self-rule."

MARK: That is an important principle, and is particularly prized in a country like the United States with its emphasis on individual freedoms, such as freedom of speech and religion.

LARRY: But, on the other hand, there is also the **principle of beneficence** which says that people, or even the government, are justified in restricting the liberty of individuals without their consent in order to prevent harm to themselves or others. Beneficence makes it our duty to benefit or protect others when we can. Obviously, it has a long history in the medical ethics tradition. It's analogous to the way a parent should look after a child, trying to keep her from harm even if it sometimes prevents her from doing what she wants.

CAROL: That's why behaving in accordance with the principle of beneficence is sometimes called 'paternalistic' behavior.

MARIA: Most laws are based on it. Seat belt laws and smoking restrictions, to name two, are based on the idea that the benefits of the principle of beneficence outweigh the principle of autonomy. And, of course, laws against crimes like rape, murder, assault, illustrate how beneficence must sometimes take precedence over autonomy.

MARK: Every society has arguments about which principle should take precedence on different issues, such as pornography and freedom of speech.

CAROL: It's also relevant to the abortion debate. I guess the main question is: "What are the justifiable limits to freedom?"

LARRY: Both principles allude to the answer: one's freedom should be limited when harm will result to others or oneself. Of course, people may disagree on the nature or extent of any alleged harm.

MARIA: That's basically why, Larry, you think that it's normally justifiable to prevent a teenager from committing suicide?

LARRY: That's part of it. The other part has to do with what we just discussed. In order to exercise autonomy one has to be a rational agent, and it does seem reasonable to think that others have the right to restrict liberty due to a lack of mental competence. Clearly, there would be harm to the suicidal teenager and her family if we allowed her to take her own life.

MARK: That's what Carol and I said earlier.

LARRY: I know. I agree with you up to that point. But, when it comes to a mentally competent adult who is terminally ill, enduring intolerable suffering, I believe the principle of autonomy outweighs the principle of beneficence. That person's autonomy ought to be respected. His desire to die should be acted upon. As I argued earlier, if it's morally permissible to respect a person's desire to refuse treatment, then it's also morally permissible to do the same and actively kill the patient.

CAROL: But what's so different about this kind of case?

MARIA: Let me answer, Larry. The difference is that there would be little or no harm resulting from active euthanasia. I mean, the patient wants to die and won't view the action as harmful. The family would also typically be involved in the long decision making process. No harm will come to them. Of course, they will be sad about the death of their loved one, but there is also a sense of relief that the loved one is no longer suffering.

LARRY: Exactly.

MARK: Well, you may be right, but remember the problems with determining mental competence and rationality?

LARRY: Sure, but you have to admit that it's not quite like your typical case of an impetuous irrational suicide.

MARK: I suppose not.

6. Immortality and Euthanasia

CAROL: You may be right, Larry, if it weren't for the issue of immortality.

LARRY: What?

CAROL: Well, if you believe that life on Earth is a preparation for the next life, then what we do here may matter greatly to one's eternal future. For example, if a person commits suicide or a doctor aids a patient by doing the job for him, what does this mean spiritually? How does God view such acts and are they detrimental to one's chance at eternal happiness in heaven?

LARRY: Are you saying that patients or doctors who do such things will automatically go to Hell?

CAROL: I don't know, but it might make a difference. After all, perhaps the suffering is meant to serve a greater purpose that God has in mind. It would be wrong to intervene.

LARRY: That sounds like a cruel God to me. Are you saying that God is *causing* the patient to suffer so that some greater good will result?

CAROL: No. God *allows* some evils, such as pain and misery, foreseeing that they can lead to a greater good in a way that we cannot always fully understand.

MARK: I have a real problem with that. Why is it morally permissible for God to allow such misery and evil to exist, especially when you believe that God is also omnipotent, omniscient, and all-good?

LARRY: And, again, as we discussed earlier, what would be the moral difference between God causing the suffering and God allowing the suffering? I still don't see it.

CAROL: Good questions, but do we really want to get into the so-called "problem of evil"?

MARK: I guess not, but I think that it's a serious problem for theism.

LARRY: Me too. At least it is for the Western conception of God.

MARK: Sure, but I still can't help but wonder why life on Earth is so sacred and important to you theists, Carol.

CAROL: What do you mean? As I've said, life is a precious gift from God and it's a preparation for eternal life.

MARK: But why do think that a few more days on Earth matters so much? If you are right, then this life is just a drop in the bucket compared to eternity. So why are you so opposed to euthanasia? Why do you even view death as such a terrible evil if it's only a transition to a "better place"?

CAROL: I see your point, but I thought that I already gave my answers to those questions.

MARK: I guess so, but it would seem to me that an atheist, such as myself, should value this life even more than you since we don't believe in anything beyond it.

MARIA: Interesting. I've often thought about that. I'm inclined to agree with you, Mark, at least to the extent that many of us who do believe in immortality may also believe that death is not always worse than prolonged suffering.

CAROL: Well, let's go on.

MARIA: Good idea. What next?

7. The Slippery Slope

MARK: I said earlier that there might be some rare individual cases where active euthanasia could be morally justified, but I'd really like to get to the heart of my opposition to it, especially to the prospect of legalizing it in this country.

MARIA: Sure. What is it?

MARK: You're all familiar with the so-called **slippery slope argument**?

LARRY: Of course.

CAROL: Yes, and I agree that we must take it very seriously.

MARIA: Me too, but why don't you explain it anyway, Mark?

MARK: Sure. The basic idea is that once we accept a certain questionable practice in some cases, we have stepped onto a slippery slope which will inevitably result in the practice of something much worse in the future. In this case, if we legalize the killing of patients in great agony who request death, we will eventually go on to accept and legalize euthanasia in increasingly more questionable circumstances. Therefore, we shouldn't take that all-important dangerous first step.

CAROL: I share your concerns, Mark. The problem is that if we start out by legalizing, say, voluntary active euthanasia for terminally ill patients, then sooner or later we will end up with nonvoluntary euthanasia for non-terminally ill patients. So why open such a Pandora's box? When a government legalizes something, it gives it kind of tacit approval and there will always be people who will want to push it further and further until we end up in a disastrous situation.

MARK: Right. I like to think of it as what is generally the best rule for a society to follow, perhaps more like a Kantian or rule-utilitarian. Even if there are some individual cases where active voluntary euthanasia would lead to the elimination of suffering with no clear negative consequences, it would still be wrong to start down that path. Acting in accordance with such a rule will eventually lead to far more negatives than positives, even if the initial intentions are good.

LARRY: But what evidence do you have for such a claim?

CAROL: Well, how about legalized abortion in this country?

MARK: Right. When abortion was first legalized, most people thought it would only be used in relatively rare cases, such as rape or incest, and perhaps there would also be some other first trimester abortions. Within twenty-five years there were a million and a half abortions per year; people had them because the parents want a boy and not a girl, some women just used it as a form of birth control, and so on. Similarly, it would be all downhill if we started allowing some cases of euthanasia.

MARIA: But can't we go back and fix it if most of us believe that it's out of hand?

MARK: Maybe, but it's not so easy. Once something is accepted and legalized in a society, it's very difficult to go back up the slippery slope. Look again at the abortion situation: now we have to struggle just to outlaw late term abortions.

MARIA: That's true. So you don't think we should start down the road in the first place?

MARK: Right. So to put it more formally, the **slippery slope**

argument says that if we accept practice A, it will eventually lead to plainly unacceptable practices X, Y, and Z. *Therefore*, we should not accept A.

It's related to the so-called **reductio ad absurdum** line of argument: Suppose that statement p is true; show that p leads to an absurd or unacceptable conclusion; *therefore*, p is false. As you know, this is a common way to argue: assume that your opponent's position is true, show how it leads to a serious problem, and then we should conclude that the original supposition is false. Remember this from yesterday?

LARRY: Yes, but shouldn't we judge the ethical rightness or wrongness of the initial practice on its own merits without becoming paranoid about what horrible things *might* follow?

MARK: Sure, but the long term consequences of doing something are relevant to its rightness or wrongness. Don't you agree?

LARRY: I guess so. That's generally in the utilitarian spirit, but we shouldn't forget that the slippery slope argument is sometimes even treated as a logical fallacy in logic textbooks. However, it still does seem to have some force. People use that type of argument against cloning research, genetic engineering, homosexual marriage, and other controversial matters.

MARK: Right, not to mention other examples from the past, such as the increase of violence and sex on television. Once we started, it was all downhill.

MARIA: But isn't using the slippery argument implying a very pessimistic view about human nature and our ability to guard against abuses?

MARK: Perhaps, but I'd prefer to call it 'realistic' instead of 'pessimistic.' And, again, it's based on past experience, so I don't think that it is some kind of unjustified paranoid fear. If anything, I think that those who don't take the slippery slope seriously enough, Larry, are too optimistic to the point of being naive.

LARRY: Really? That's the first time I've been called 'naive.'

CAROL: I have to agree with Mark, although I hate to think so negatively about human nature. I just think we need to be very careful whenever we start down such a dangerous road.

LARRY: Well, I don't think I'm naive. You should see some of the criminals I defend as part of my job. However, we do also need to be careful not to be paralyzed into inaction so that we never make important changes in social policy and the law. Some changes are for the better and we need to try to figure out honestly which ones are and which ones aren't. Someone may always cry "look out for the slippery slope," but I'd like to hear more about what would be so terrible if we legalized active voluntary euthanasia. I'm optimistic that we could design a system to guard against potential abuses. For example, in Holland, active voluntary euthanasia is an available option, but certain important conditions must be met.

MARK: Well, I'm not optimistic. We can discuss Holland later, but I think that it's a perfect example of the slippery slope. For one thing, terminal illness is not even required there in order for one to be euthanized. Shouldn't it be a prerequisite?

LARRY: Maybe, although there could be some cases where it shouldn't be; for example, a paraplegic or a severely burned person who can be kept alive indefinitely.

MARK: But how close to death does one have to be in order to count as 'terminally ill'?

MARIA: How about three months?

MARK: Fine, but that's arbitrary. Do you really think it would stay at three months?

LARRY: Why not?

CAROL: Well, I'm sure we'd immediately see law suits on behalf of patients who have four months left, and then five months left, etc. Where will it end? That's the problem. Even if it doesn't start out that way, sooner or later 'terminally ill' will come mean almost anything.

MARK: Right.

LARRY: I don't agree. Don't you think that we are smart and rational enough to keep that from happening?

MARK: No. As I said earlier, our track record is not very good. I'd like to think we are so rational that we could carefully guard against these problems, but the historical evidence doesn't support that view.

CAROL: I agree, and it's not just the so-called "average person" who might start to slide down the slippery slope. It's also just as clear that the supposedly 'intellectual' of our society do it all the time. College professors, lawyers, doctors, the courts, and Congresspersons are just as much to blame when a society slides down a slippery slope, despite our claims to be so much more rational than the average person.

MARIA: Well, I'd like to think we can do better, but I agree that the slippery slope is a compelling reason to be very careful about how, or if, we should legalize euthanasia in this country.

LARRY: I still don't see the compelling argument against legalizing it with careful guidelines. Can you get more specific, Mark, about what you think would happen if, say, active voluntary euthanasia were legalized?

MARK: Sure. I've already mentioned the problem with defining terminal illness, not to mention the problem with mental competence. The evidence from Holland is also starting to show how we could get to a point of "euthanasia on demand" much in the way that we now basically have abortion on demand in this country. For example, the amount of pain or suffering really doesn't have to be so great anymore. And the slide from voluntary to nonvoluntary euthanasia is also well on its way. Euthanasia is now routinely performed on patients without their consent.

LARRY: I'm not so sure about that. I'd have to see some of the data you are relying on.

MARK: Sure, but it would be even worse in a larger country such as ours, where we have a much greater number of elderly and a more complex economic and insurance system.

LARRY: Perhaps.

MARK: Well, let me just list another group of potential problems and abuses:

(1) There would be reduced pressure to find cures or relieve symptoms.

(2) There would be pressure on many patients, who already feel like a burden, to request euthanasia and relieve their families of the financial and other burdens of prolonged care. This would also aid the slide from voluntary to nonvoluntary euthanasia.

(3) There would be a greater likelihood of giving up too early. We don't want patients abandoning hope at the very time they most need to fight for their lives. And, also, doctors do make mistakes in diagnosis.

(4) Whether or not one believes, as I do, that killing patients is contrary to what the medical profession stands for, euthanasia would carry with it a psychological burden that doctors shouldn't have to carry. As it is, doctors suffer from higher than normal rates of alcoholism, depression, and marital problems.

(5) There is the general danger and inevitable consequence of the cheapening of human life. Think of the message we would be sending our children. Again, I would point to the parallel with abortion here.

(6) With the growing concern over medical costs, euthanasia would be a cheap solution. Pressure would mount to use it instead of more costly ways to preserve life.

(7) There would be an increased fear of hospital and doctors. As it is, people don't like to go to the doctor or the hospital, but legalizing euthanasia would heighten that fear to the point of losing trust in doctors who should only be in the business of saving and curing people. Many preventable deaths would therefore result from such fears.

MARIA: Wow! That's some list. I can see how many of them might come to pass, although I'm not entirely convinced. They are genuine risks, but you make it sound like they'll inevitably occur.

MARK: Yes, again, based on past experience, the evidence from

Holland's system, and knowledge of human nature. But I don't see why the burden of proof falls on me.

LARRY: How do you mean?

MARK: Well, the question is: should we gamble with legalizing euthanasia despite the risks? It seems to me that those of you who answer yes should carry the burden of explaining why each of these abuses will not occur. I mean, why take such a chance?

LARRY: Well, I don't think all of your concerns would come to pass, but even if they did, I don't think they would be so serious as to outweigh the benefits of legalized euthanasia. Even if I grant you that there will be *some* abuse, you need to show that the negative consequences would outweigh the benefits.

MARK: What benefits?

LARRY: Well, for example, the relief of unnecessary suffering on the part of both patient and family, and the peace of mind that we'd each have knowing that we have that option.

MARK: But I don't see how those would outweigh all of the problems that I have listed, especially in the long run. As I said, I think that the burden is on you to show otherwise.

LARRY: Well, I'm not sure why, but let's drop it here.

MARK: Sure.

CAROL: Fine, but I did just want to remind you that we haven't spent very much time on cases involving infants, which would have to be classified as nonvoluntary, whether they are passive or active. Many of Mark's slippery slope concerns apply here as well. And perhaps it would even be worse, since a severely deformed or ill infant cannot speak for herself. The temptation would be dangerously strong, for example, to save medical costs or for parents not to want such an "abnormal child" if euthanasia were legalized.

MARK: Yes. There is the danger of just getting rid of such children merely upon the parents request. We would start to weed out the "undesirables" and the "abnormal." What kind of society treats its less fortunate in such a way? It almost starts to sounds like Nazi Germany.

CAROL: Right. We would start by letting severely deformed terminally ill infants die, but then end up actively killing infants with less severe conditions such as Down's Syndrome or some minor physical abnormality.

LARRY: Maybe, but I doubt it. And, anyway, I don't think that all cases of euthanasia on defective infants would be wrong. As it is, passive euthanasia on severely deformed infants occurs every day, so why keep all active euthanasia illegal?

MARK: Well, again, for the slippery slope reasons I've explained to you.

CAROL: Not to mention some of the more religious reasons I expressed earlier.

LARRY: I still think that the principle of autonomy must take priority here, but perhaps we've reached a stalemate at this point.

8. Assisted Suicide

MARIA: Maybe we'd be better off only legalizing assisted suicide instead of active euthanasia. In a case of assisted suicide the patient ultimately kills herself, although it is with the help of a doctor or someone else.

MARK: Why do you think that would be better?

MARIA: For one thing, it would eliminate one of your earlier main concerns about active euthanasia; namely, that it's wrong to have doctors actively causing the death of patients.

MARK: Sure, but doctors helping patients to die seems almost as bad to me. From a Kantian point of view, I have some real problems with the morality of suicide in general, and many of the same slippery slope problems still arise with regard to assisted suicide. Look at Jack Kevorkian: Many of us have been rather nervous about having someone like him as the champion of this cause.

CAROL: I agree, Mark. And, from a religious point of view, I believe that committing suicide is just as wrong as active euthanasia.

LARRY: As you might guess, I think that assisted suicide can be morally right in some circumstances. I know that I'd like to have that option if I were ever in such a horrible situation.

MARIA: But don't you think it matters to what degree the doctor assists the patient?

LARRY: What do you mean?

MARIA: Well, there are basically three possible types of assistance differing in the degree of doctor involvement: (1) *providing information* to the patient so that suicide can be achieved in the least traumatic and most effective manner, (2) *providing the means* necessary when the suicidal person would otherwise be without such means; for example, bringing a lethal dose to the patient, and (3) *directly aiding and supervising the suicide*, such as mixing a lethal dose of drugs and holding it to the patient's lips or setting up a lethal injection so that the patient only has to press a button to release the drug into the bloodstream. Let's call them 'level-one,' 'level-two,' and 'level-three.'

LARRY: I think that all three would be morally permissible under certain conditions. Since I believe that some cases of active euthanasia would be morally permissible, then I naturally would morally accept assisted suicide in those cases.

MARIA: Sure, but one might oppose active euthanasia for the slippery slope reasons we saw earlier, but be in favor of some form of assisted suicide.

MARK: I guess so. Is that partly because you think assisted suicide would eliminate some of the slippery slope concerns?

MARIA: Yes, there would be less chance of abuse; for example, it should all but eliminate your concerns about giving doctors the power to kill, killing patients without their consent, and the slide from voluntary to nonvoluntary.

MARK: Maybe assisted suicide would have fewer potential abuses than active euthanasia, but too many would still remain. We should keep it illegal. I suppose that if we did legalize it, I would at most support level-one. Helping someone to gain access to the information may not be wrong, but anyone could do that. Books are currently available for that purpose. So, in a sense, it is already legal. But doctors would not have to be involved, whereas levels-two and three seem to require doctor assistance.

MARIA: I see. I think that level-two might also be morally permissible in some cases, but perhaps we should avoid legalizing it up through level-three. I share your slippery slope concerns for level-three, and that was the level of assistance provided by Kevorkian.

LARRY: What was so wrong with what he did?

MARK: For one thing, he didn't even seem to know his patients very well. I also didn't trust his motives. He seemed to have a morbid fascination with death. After all, he was a pathologist. Everyone called him "doctor," which he was, but few seem to know about what kind of doctor he was and the fact that he was retired. Even though he was frequently acquitted of criminal charges, it was important that we had the option of charging him with a crime. Just imagine what he would have done if assisted suicide were legal!

LARRY: But why didn't *the families* of his dead patients take him to court?

MARK: I don't know.

LARRY: I think it was because they didn't think he was doing anything wrong. That has to mean something.

CAROL: Well, I can't morally accept any of the three levels of assistance. Perhaps we can try to understand why someone would commit suicide under certain horrible conditions. Perhaps we shouldn't even stop such a person from committing suicide, as opposed to the way that we normally would intervene to prevent a suicide. But there is a big moral difference between saying "I won't stop you" and "I will help you." I don't think we should ever go beyond the former to the latter.

MARK: Interesting, I guess it would be the difference between respecting the person's autonomy and agreeing with what that person is about to do.

CAROL: Yes, it's the difference between respect and assent.

MARIA: Well, let's end it for today. I need to go up to my room and call home.

CAROL: I have to go too. I'm participating in a discussion panel in the morning.

LARRY: Okay, but just remember that I don't think assisted suicide would be enough. We also need active euthanasia for those who cannot kill themselves. Some illnesses and disabilities don't allow a patient to kill himself; for example, severe paralysis or the final weakened stages of many diseases.

MARIA: On that happy note, I'll see you tomorrow. How about we go out for lunch?

LARRY: Good idea. There's an excellent restaurant across the street. Let's meet there around noon.

CAROL: Sure.

MARK: Sounds good.

THE THIRD DAY

ABORTION

AFTER LUNCH

After having lunch at a nearby restaurant, they walk back to the hotel and find comfortable chairs near the hotel lobby. They each have a cup of coffee purchased from a hotel coffee stand.

1. The Law

MARK: What's wrong, Carol? You look distracted.

CAROL: I'm fine, but I just can't get off my mind this morning's discussion panel. As I mentioned to you at lunch, I thought it went well but I wish there was more time to address the arguments more completely.

MARIA: Well, there's no time like the present.

CAROL: As you all know, I believe that virtually all cases of abortion are morally wrong. After all, it involves the killing of a human being.

LARRY: I couldn't disagree with you more.

MARK: I know that I'll agree more with Carol. I'm also pro-life.

MARIA: Well, I'd consider myself pro-choice, but probably not to Larry's extent.

LARRY: If we're going to discuss this topic, shouldn't we first be clear about the law in the United States so that we can debate as to whether it should be changed for any ethical reasons?

CAROL: Of course, but we should also make explicit some of the basic biological facts of fetal development. People often just seem to ignore them.

MARK: Yes.

MARIA: Well, it's currently legal for a woman to have an abortion. Since the 1973 seven-to-two *Roe v. Wade* Supreme Court decision, the right to an abortion has been considered a Constitutional right in the eyes of the law. Under the fictitious name of Jane Roe, a single pregnant woman challenged the constitutionality of the existing Texas criminal abortion law. At the time, in Texas, the performance of an abortion except to save the life of the pregnant woman was illegal and carried with it a prison term of two to five years.

LARRY: Right, but States also do have a legitimate interest in protecting the health of the pregnant woman; for example, to ensure safe abortions. The State may also have a legitimate interest in protecting fetal life, but not until after the point of viability; that is, the point at which the fetus could live outside the mother's womb. This is usually at about twenty-eight weeks. So States can and do outlaw late-term or third trimester abortions with some rare exceptions.

MARK: But the sad result has been that abortion was made legal virtually *on demand*; that is, for any reason at all up through at least the sixth month of pregnancy. What a disastrous decision for the unborn. In this case, I think that the current law is unethical.

MARIA: Well, I agree with you that abortions *for some reasons and at some times* are wrong, especially from, say, the fourth month on. However, I think that the *Roe v. Wade* decision was important for respecting the autonomy of women and that early abortions are not morally wrong. Women should have the right to choose.

CAROL: Please don't speak on my behalf as a woman. I don't think anyone has the right to kill their own child, whether it's before or after birth.

LARRY: But is a fetus a *child*? Why do you insist on calling it one?

CAROL: Because it has most of the same biological features as a child. Why do you insist on calling it a "fetus"? Is that how expecting parents usually talk about their unborn children? I don't think so.

LARRY: As you know, 'fetus' is the proper prenatal biological term. But you call it what you want and I'll call it what I want.

CAROL: Fine, but this already shows how even just the use of language can color the discussion.

LARRY: Sure, but anyway, the Supreme Court basically ruled that the "unborn" are not covered when the terms "person" and "citizen" are used in the Constitution; for example, in the Fourteenth Amendment's mention of not "depriving any *person* of life, liberty, or property, without due process of law." Moreover, the Court ruled that a Constitutionally recognized right to privacy is broad enough to include a woman's decision of whether or not to terminate her pregnancy.

MARK: Well, it's amazing how they just made up such a right to privacy. The Constitution does not explicitly mention any right of privacy, and especially not to that extent. As for the business about "persons" and "citizens," it is true that the unborn are not citizens in the usual sense of the term, but the Court seems to have arbitrarily stipulated what counts as a "person."

CAROL: Right, first they say that even though there is no explicit mention of a right to privacy, it still covers a woman's right to choose an abortion. But then they say that since the unborn are not explicitly mentioned as part of the meaning of 'person' or 'citizen,' they are *not* covered under the Fourteenth Amendment. I don't get it.

MARK: Me either.

MARIA: Well, they didn't just decide the case without any historical basis. Read their decision again and you'll see that they cite many historical cases which serve as a basis for the decision.

LARRY: Right, and the bottom line is that the unborn have never been recognized in the law as persons in the whole sense.

CAROL: Well, maybe, but again this is a case where I believe that the law is wrong. It's just like slavery. For many years blacks and even women were also not considered to be "persons in the whole sense" until we finally realized how wrong that was. The same applies here as far as I'm concerned. We can't just pick and choose arbitrarily which human beings "count" as persons. It's a license to oppress and kill those who fall outside the definition. We should protect all human life equally.

LARRY: That's a terrible analogy.

CAROL: Why?

LARRY: Because women and blacks were discriminated against even though they shared with us the most important feature of being a person; for example, self-consciousness and rationality. Fetuses do not have those features. And a fetus is inside the woman's body and can't be compared to the historical biases against women and minorities.

MARK: Sure, but fetuses are now being killed and discriminated against even though they share with us the biological fact that they are living human beings with all of the same biological features.

MARIA: But what sorts of biological features do you have in mind?

2. Fetal Development

MARK: Well, let's look at fetal development. Even the early fertilized egg or ovum contains a full genetic code. The **zygote** then travels through the fallopian tube and is implanted into the uterine wall at about two weeks.

CAROL: Right, and then it's technically called an **embryo** for about the next six weeks. During that time, the circulatory system begins to develop, the heart begins to beat, and most body parts are forming, such as the head, hands, and feet.

MARK: And then the **fetus**, as it is technically called from about the eighth week until birth, continues to grow and develop. It grows from about two inches to much larger, along with the continued development of the eyes and bones. Some brain waves are detected as early as eight weeks. Hearing is clearly present at about five months. And then **quickening**, as you know, is the point at which the woman begins to feel the movements of the fetus, usually from about the sixteenth week on. Often, however, the term 'fetus' is used to cover all three stages of development.

MARIA: We know all that, but despite some physical similarities to us late in fetal development, it's still clear that the fetus is not very similar to us at the earlier stages, especially in the first two months or so when it is a zygote or embryo. For one thing, it's not even conscious at all. How could we possibly ethically or legally justify viewing them as having the same rights as us?

CAROL: Well, at any stage, it's a living human being. That should be enough.

LARRY: So you mean 'human being' in some genetic sense. Right?

CAROL: Sure.

LARRY: And what about the term 'living'?

CAROL: What do you mean? Of course the fetus is *alive*. It's a developing biological organism with living cells and tissue. That can't be denied. Are we now going to redefine the word 'alive' so that fetuses are not alive?

MARIA: Of course not, but the issue is the moral status of a fetus.

CAROL: Fine, but the fetus has living cells. It even has a heart beat.

LARRY: Sure.

MARK: And that's why it's obviously true that a child, or something human, is killed during every abortion. I mean, all you have to do is look at some of those gruesome pictures of aborted fetuses. The abortion procedures just turn my stomach. I can't believe that we let this happen in our country over four thousand times a day. It's a contemporary holocaust.

MARIA: Clever appeal to emotion, but that doesn't really settle very much. And pictures of aborted *embryos* are not so "gruesome."

MARK: Perhaps not, but don't you show pictures of killed and tortured animals in order to influence opinion in the animal rights debate?

MARIA: Sure, but can't we hold off on that until tomorrow?

MARK: Yes, but don't accuse me of emotionalism unless you are also prepared to accept blame yourself. My point is only that when we really see what happens in an abortion, it shows exactly how human fetuses are before they are killed so mercilessly. Every woman and man should see pictures of fetal development, so that we at least have all the information before ignorantly calling fetuses "globs of tissue." That's certainly not the way that *happy* pregnant women think of them.

CAROL: Here are some of the ugly facts. Abortionists usually use uterine aspiration for early abortions: the fetus is sucked out of the uterus by means of a tube connected to a suction pump. In later abortions, a forceps is used to dismember the fetus in the uterus; the remains of the fetus are then withdrawn through the cervix. Also, the fetus is sometimes first killed with an injection of saline solution, which induces labor thereby expelling the fetus. The unborn child is, in essence, burned to death. What's going on here?

MARIA: Well, I am familiar with abortion methods and with fetal development. I have two kids, remember?

CAROL: Yes.

LARRY: So merely being familiar with fetal development does not automatically translate into agreement with your position, Carol.

CAROL: I know, and I'm amazed that it doesn't.

LARRY: But there are so many other issues: the concept of a person, the comparative rights of the woman and the fetus, the woman's right to choose, the right to privacy, and so on. You make it sound so simple.

3. Genetic Humans versus Persons

CAROL: As far as I'm concerned, it is fairly simple. I can think of an argument with two premises and a conclusion that summarizes it for me.

MARIA: What is it?

CAROL:

(1) It is wrong to kill innocent human beings.
(2) Fetuses are innocent human beings.
Therefore, (3) It is wrong to kill fetuses.

MARIA: That's a bit too simple.

CAROL: Why? It makes sense to me. And notice that I included the word 'innocent' in premise 1 in order to allow that cases of self-defense can be morally right. Also, although I oppose capital punishment, someone who is in favor of it could still accept premise 1.

MARIA: Sure, but the problem is that you commit **the fallacy of equivocation**; that is, you are using a single term or expression with *two* different meanings. You can't do that.

CAROL: How do you mean? Which expression?

MARIA: 'Human being.' In order for both of your premises to be clearly acceptable, you have to mean something different by 'human being' in each premise. We must remember to distinguish between 'human' in *the genetic sense* of the term and 'human' in *the psychological sense*. Only the latter is what we mean by a 'person'; that is, a person is best defined as someone who has the following features: (1) consciousness, (2) reasoning ability, (3) self-motivated or voluntary activity, (4) the ability to communicate, and (5) self-consciousness. There clearly could be non-human persons, such as alien beings, or human non-persons, such as comatose vegetables. So clearly the class of humans and the class of persons are not identical.

LARRY: Right. Let's agree to use the terms in that way and distinguish genetic humans, or members of our biological species *Homo Sapien*, from persons in the psychological sense.

CAROL: Fine, although I'm not so sure about your list of features. But go on.

MARIA: Well, the only way that both of your premises are uncontroversially true is if you mean 'person' by 'human being' in premise 1 and if you mean 'genetic human' by 'human being' in premise 2. That should be rather obvious. I think everyone would agree that it's always wrong to kill an innocent *person*, and it's equally clear that fetuses are *genetically* human. But, of course, by equivocating in this way, your conclusion does not follow from the premises.

LARRY: And, Carol, if you keep the meaning of 'human being' the same in both premises, then one of them would be false, or at least question begging.

CAROL: How so?

LARRY: If you mean the 'person' or psychological sense of 'human being' throughout the argument, then premise 1 is true but premise 2 is clearly false. Fetuses do not have any of the five traits of a person for the first few months and, at most, only have some primitive form of consciousness for the remainder of the nine months.

On the other hand, if you mean the genetic sense throughout, then premise 2 is obviously true, but premise 1 simply begs the question; that is, it assumes what you are trying to prove. You can't try to prove that it's wrong to kill fetuses by using the premise that it's wrong to kill all innocent genetic humans. I mean, the whole issue here is whether or not it's *always* wrong to kill a genetic human.

CAROL: But I do believe that it's always wrong to kill an innocent genetic human.

MARIA: Fine, but you then need to give some independent support for your claim in premise 1. And any reason you give will likely be rejected by someone who is pro-choice. You will not have gained any ground. For one thing, simply calling abortion 'murder' isn't enough. As you know, not all cases of killing are murders. For example, you mentioned self-defense, which is a killing that isn't a murder. The term 'murder' carries with it the connotation of *wrongful* or *unjustifiable* killing. And so you need to give some independent reason for why killing, in the case of abortion, is wrong.

CAROL: Sure, but we may just get to a point where we hold very different views on these fundamental matters. For me, it's mostly based on religion. For others, like Mark, perhaps not. But the fact remains that abortion involves the killing of an innocent human being. That should be enough to show that it's wrong.

4. Potential versus Actual Persons

MARK: I suppose it comes down to the question "What sorts of things have a strong right to life?" We need to decide, for ethical and legal reasons, what kinds of living things a society ought to protect against being killed. On this point, I agree much more with Carol even if her initial argument fails as it stands. Fetuses ought to be protected against being killed, first, because they are human beings and human life is intrinsically valuable. Second, and more important, although fetuses are not *actual* persons they are *potential* persons. It's very likely that each fetus will become a person just like you and me, as long as it is properly nourished. That's how all of us started out; sometimes I think people forget that.

LARRY: But why should *potentiality* carry so much moral weight?

MARK: Because it coheres with the view that fetuses are precious and unique potential people. I think what most bothers pro-lifers is that with *each* abortion a unique and distinct human individual is killed. There will never again be one like him or her. It's no different than a young child being killed, and everyone seems so horrified when a child is murdered. The agonizing sense of "what might have been" is very much the same. And unlike any other part of a pregnant woman's body, the fetus is a genetically distinct potential person.

MARIA: Well, the difference between a two-month-old fetus and a two-month-old infant is enormous. And how can you be sure that a fetus will develop into a person? It's not certain.

CAROL: No, but it's very highly likely as long as the fetus is properly nourished, especially after implantation into the uterine wall. Of course it's not guaranteed, but why should that matter? There's no guarantee that a two-year-old will reach adulthood, but is that a reason in favor of killing it?

MARIA: Of course not.

MARK: Maybe we should make it clear that 'potentiality,' in this discussion, is not just some vague possibility. It's a high probability, and the main factor is simply time. The fetus gradually develops; it grows both physically and psychologically. To snuff out a life at any of its early stages is clearly wrong for the same reason that it's wrong to kill you or me: it deprives that fetus or child of a valuable future like ours. Killing the fetus deprives it of all future experiences and activities. That's the same reason why it's wrong to kill you. Aside from the negative affects that it will have on your loved ones, killing you now would deprive you of your future life. And that's what makes it wrong.

MARIA: Interesting, but an early fetus is not even conscious. It's not as if it would be missing anything; for example, it doesn't have any goals in life or desires to do anything.

MARK: But why must an organism actually have conscious desires or goals in order to be protected against being killed? Again, it's just a matter of time. I would put it by saying that it is clearly not *in the interest of the fetus* for it be killed, whether or not it's aware of its own life yet.

MARIA: I don't see how a nonconscious organism can have any "interests" at all, but go on.

MARK: Anyway, we could revise Carol's argument without even mentioning genetic humans:

> (1) It is wrong to kill innocent actual or potential persons.
> (2) Fetuses are innocent potential persons.
> *Therefore*, (3) It is wrong to kill fetuses.

CAROL: That's fine with me.

MARIA: But aren't you saying something like "since the fetus potentially has a right to life, then it actually has a right to life"? If so, that's a terrible argument.

CAROL: Why?

MARIA: It's fallacious in the same way that one couldn't validly argue that "since a fetus or child potentially has a right to vote, then it actually has a right to vote."

CAROL: I see, but I don't think pro-lifers are making that logical error. We're not saying that potentially having x entails actually having x. We're instead arguing that since x is *potentially a person*, x *actually has a right to life*. That's very different and doesn't commit any logical fallacy.

MARK: Right, and so the basic claim is: any entity that is actually or potentially a person has a strong right to life.

LARRY: I don't agree at all, and I want to raise another objection to your reliance on potentiality.

MARK: Sure.

LARRY: Doesn't your view entail that all contraception is wrong? After all, doesn't using contraception often prevent a person from existing in the same way that abortions do? Where do you draw the line and how can you justify contraception if you are pro-life?

CAROL: Actually, I do believe that contraception is wrong for various religious reasons. However, I don't see that the wrongness of contraception follows from the wrongness of abortion.

MARK: I think there's a big difference between contraception and abortion, except perhaps for those forms of contraception, such as IUD's, that allow fertilization and then cause the destruction of the fertilized egg. But, in any case, it is only *after conception* that there's a single individual existing thing that is a potential person. Sperm and eggs are not, *separately or individually*, potential persons. For example, we can't point to a single sperm and truthfully say "that is a potential person." On the other hand, the fertilized egg is a potential person.

LARRY: I suppose so, but it's still not that simple. Just because there isn't a single potential person before conception, there would still often be two individuals immediately before conception, a sperm and the egg, prevented from uniting into a potential person. I'm still not sure why you think that wouldn't be wrong.

MARK: Well, conception is the best non-arbitrary point to draw the line. Any time earlier, as you said, there would be two individuals. There would be no single subject that would be killed if those cells are prevented from uniting. But an abortion ends the life of a single subject.

LARRY: I'll let you slide on this. Let me think about it some more.

MARK: Sure.

MARIA: But pro-lifers must acknowledge that actual persons have a right to life.

CAROL: Of course.

MARIA: So then what about when a pregnant woman's life is at stake? Isn't abortion morally permissible under those conditions?

MARK: I think so.

CAROL: Me too.

MARIA: But then aren't you really admitting that the pregnant woman's rights carry more moral weight than the fetus' rights?

MARK: Not generally. Pro-lifers will say that an actual person's *right to life* outweighs a potential person's right to life. But this only allows for the abortion exception when the woman's *life* is at stake. Virtually all pro-lifers agree on this, but these abortions account for less than one-percent of abortions.

CAROL: Right. We're talking about cases where the woman's life is really at stake, not just any possible health risk associated with pregnancy. There are many of those, but I don't think any of them should outweigh the child's right to life.

MARIA: Why not? Childbirth can be dangerous and carrying a child for nine-months can involve many health considerations short of death.

CAROL: Of course, but the child's right to life must outweigh what usually only involves some relatively minor discomfort or illness. How can you compare?

MARK: The key point is that not just *any* of the rights of a pregnant woman can outweigh the child's right to life. Only the woman's right to life would. But as we all know, women have abortions for reasons that don't even approach such a level; for example, having the child will "interfere" with the perceived happiness of the woman, say, financially or career-wise.

CAROL: To take a life for any of those reasons is selfish and irresponsible in the first place. And men are equally to blame. They often act irresponsibly when they get women pregnant or they leave the woman to deal with the problem herself. She feels alone, without support, and is overwhelmed by the circumstances. I understand the predicament, but abortion is not the answer. It's the wrong path to take.

LARRY: I want to return to the question "What has a right to life?"

and explain my view. I couldn't disagree more with Mark and Carol.

MARK: Go on.

LARRY: I believe that all and only people, *actual* people, have a right to life. And, again, a person is someone with the five characteristics we mentioned earlier: (1) consciousness, (2) reasoning ability, (3) self-motivated or voluntary behavior, (4) the ability to communicate, and (5) self-consciousness.

CAROL: Must an organism have all five in order to be a person?

LARRY: Well, I'd have to say that at least reasoning and some form of consciousness are necessary. And certainly the ability to reason and self-consciousness are sufficient for being a person. Again, clearly some human beings are not persons; for example, someone in an irreversible coma. And if an organism had none of the five characteristics and someone called it a 'person,' we should say that he didn't understand the meaning of "person" or that he is confusing 'person' with some genetic concept.

CAROL: So you don't think that even a late term fetus has a right to life?

LARRY: That's right. It's not a person, and I remain unconvinced by your emphasis on potentiality. Therefore, I believe that abortions can be morally permissible all through pregnancy.

CAROL: For any reason and at whatever stage?

LARRY: Sure.

CAROL: But what about small infants? They don't, for example, have the ability to reason. Do infants have a right to life?

LARRY: No.

CAROL: What? Really? So infanticide wouldn't be a violation of a right to life?

LARRY: That's right.

MARK: It would then be morally permissible to kill infants?

LARRY: Well, put it this way: it wouldn't be murder to kill an infant. However, it doesn't necessarily follow that infanticide is morally permissible. I mean, we might think that an act is wrong without thinking that it's murder, involving a violation of a right to life. For example, other people might want to have the child even if the parents don't. This is a reason against killing a newborn. Unlike when the woman is carrying a fetus, an infant can be given to someone else who wants it. So long as there are people in this country who value infants and are willing and able to care for them, it would still be wrong to destroy them after birth.

MARK: That sounds dangerously relativistic to me. Remember our conversation on relativism? What if a society didn't value infants? Would infanticide be morally permissible in that society at that time?

LARRY: I suppose so, but I doubt that would happen.

MARK: Really? Once again, your naive optimism about human nature continues to amaze me. Perhaps a society wouldn't devalue *all* of its young because then it would probably die off, but surely a society might not value infants very much, leaving only enough infants to continue the species.

LARRY: In any case, infanticide can still be wrong without it being murder for analogous reasons to those which make it wrong to destroy works of art or natural resources.

CAROL: I can't believe what I'm hearing: comparing the value of human infants to works of art. Terrible!

LARRY: Sorry that you feel that way, but it's the truth.

MARK: But for someone sounding so relativistic, you're sure way outside of the majority in this culture. Isn't it considered murder to kill a one-month old infant in the eyes of the law?

LARRY: Sure, but I don't think it should be. No *person* is killed. But, again, I'm not saying that it's morally right to kill infants.

CAROL: Again, I can't believe what I'm hearing. Should a man get convicted of a lesser crime and receive a lesser sentence if he kills an infant? Unbelievable!! Maybe that will become the new defense tactic for those who murder infants: "well, I didn't kill *a person*."

MARK: Anyway, you're therefore not really a relativist, Larry, since you seem to be saying that the majority in our culture is wrong.

LARRY: I suppose.

MARK: And what about mentally defective human beings? Alzheimer's patients? Down's Syndrome children? Do they have a right to life?

LARRY: No, if they are not persons. To the extent that they've lost certain central features of personhood, such as rationality, they would also not have a right to life. Again, however, it may not necessarily be morally permissible to kill them. But it also wouldn't be murder.

MARK: Well, I think that the consequences of your position show how absurd it is. Any theory of rights implying that it's not murder to kill a newborn infant or a mentally defective human must be false. It's a *reductio ad absurdum*.

CAROL: Yes, and what about people who are in temporary comas or are temporarily unconscious. They are not actual persons. Do they lose their right to life, Larry?

LARRY: I don't think so.

CAROL: But why?

LARRY: Well, the lack of consciousness is temporary and they *were* persons once before. So we should wait to see if they will regain their psychological characteristics.

CAROL: So are you now saying that an organism has a right to life as long as *either* it is an actual person *or* it was a person at some point in the past?

LARRY: I suppose so, but notice that a fetus was *never* a person.

MARK: But the recently deceased or those in irreversible comas *were* persons; do they have a right to life even though they are not alive in any psychological sense?

LARRY: Of course not, but in those cases there is no chance of becoming a person again.

MARK: Oh! I see! So *the potential* to become a person is really what counts; isn't it? And the likelihood of becoming a person again in many of these cases is much lower than the likelihood of a typical fetus becoming a person. Right?

LARRY: I suppose so, but the difference is that those who are temporarily unconscious might become persons *again*, whereas a fetus was never a person.

MARK: I give up.

MARIA: I also have to reject your criterion of moral personhood, Larry. It faces too many serious objections.

LARRY: Fine, but what do you think is better?

MARIA: Well, as I said earlier, I don't believe that early abortions are morally wrong. Part of the reason is simply that early fetuses aren't conscious creatures; they're not even capable of feeling pain. Consciousness in any form is the key to this whole debate.

MARK: How do you mean?

MARIA: I think that any actually conscious creature has a right to life. So that clearly includes newborn infants and mentally defective humans, but it also includes fetuses once significant brain activity begins around the third or fourth month. Obviously there are degrees of consciousness going all the way up to rationality and self-consciousness, but that's irrelevant to having a right to life.

CAROL: So you'd oppose all abortions from, say, the fourth month on?

MARIA: Yes, unless it's to save the life of the woman. But since the vast majority of abortions are performed in the first three months, I don't have a serious problem with the current law, although clearly there are too many abortions performed every day. And there are also thousands of later term abortions that do occur and shouldn't be permitted.

LARRY: But what's wrong with the so-called "point of viability," which is now at around twenty-eight weeks?

MARIA: I don't think it can be used to distinguish morally wrong from morally permissible abortions.

LARRY: Why not?

MARIA: Well, even in the *Roe v. Wade* decision, 'viability' is defined as "being able to live outside the mother's womb, *albeit with artificial aid*." I don't think the Court should have put so much weight on it. For one thing, the point of viability can change, and has already changed, depending on the technology available to keep a fetus alive outside the womb.

CAROL: Yes, it's amazing how this has changed in the hospitals over the years. Premature babies survive now in ways that they couldn't have in the past.

MARIA: Right. My point is that viability has become and will continue to become earlier and earlier. We can even imagine a future where viability is very early in pregnancy, so that fetuses could be removed early and then developed outside the womb. Would all pro-choicers then agree that any abortion after viability would be wrong? I don't think so. And so the moral issue of abortion shouldn't rest on such a changeable and technology-dependent point in fetal development. On the other hand, becoming conscious is a much more straightforward and unchanging point in fetal development.

MARK: I see and I agree with your critique of the viability criterion, but I still think you don't take potentiality seriously enough. I mean, a couple of months or so, why should that matter for having a right to life?

MARIA: Do we have to discuss that again?

MARK: I guess not, but I'm still puzzled about your view since I know you're a strong animal rights activist.

MARIA: Puzzled about what?

MARK: Well, by your criterion, dogs and pigs have a right to life.

MARIA: Yes.

MARK: But then you must hold that it is morally permissible to kill a two-month old fetus, but virtually always wrong to kill a pig or a cat?

MARIA: That's right, but can't we discuss this some other time?

MARK: Sure, but that's one reason why I can't accept your criterion. Killing a pig is murder, but having an early abortion is not. That's almost as absurd as some of Larry's views.

MARIA: Why? I'm very consistent: all conscious life has intrinsic value and should be protected against being killed. And my view avoids Larry's problems with infants and mentally defective humans. As a matter of fact, I think that you (*pointing to Carol*) and Mark also have a problem with mentally defective humans.

CAROL: How so?

MARIA: Earlier you seemed happy with the idea that all actual or potential persons have a right to life. Remember?

CAROL: Sure.

MARIA: But a severely retarded human is not an actual or a potential person. Neither is a woman with a progressively deteriorating

Alzheimer's condition. Even your criterion seems to rule them out as having a right to life.

CAROL: Good point; that's all the more reason why we should accept the religious view that all *human* life is a gift from God. All humans, in the genetic sense, have an intrinsic right to life.

MARK: Leaving aside Carol's religious reply, remember I also said that fetuses ought to be protected against being killed just because they are human beings and human life is intrinsically valuable. This was before I even mentioned potentiality.

MARIA: Then why do you even bring in the concept of a person at all, along with the psychological traits we discussed?

MARK: Well, you and Larry rightly raised it in response to Carol's initial argument. I think it's an important aspect of this debate, and I was at that time presenting a criterion with personhood in mind. I don't see why we can't hold *both* that all innocent humans have a right to life *and* that all potential or actual persons have a right to life. So what if there's sometimes an overlap between the two?

MARIA: I see, but it sounds rather odd to have two criteria in that way.

MARK: Maybe you're right. Perhaps we can combine them in a more straightforward way.

MARIA: How?

MARK: How about this? All and only members of any species that *generally* possess the five features of personhood have a right to life, whether or not the species is *Homo Sapien* and whether or not each individual of the species is a person.

CAROL: That is probably better.

LARRY: Why?

CAROL: Well, for one thing, it avoids all of the objections we've discussed so far.

MARK: Right, it would grant a right to life to fetuses, newborns, mentally defective humans, and so on. They are members of a species which *generally* contain persons. And this criterion can also allow for persons of different species. If there are alien races of people, then they should also have a right to life. And so would their infants, mental defectives, fetuses, and so on. That's the way it should be.

MARIA: I don't agree, especially since you are not clearly including all conscious animals.

MARK: Perhaps some higher mammals should be included, but that's it.

MARIA: But why should moral personhood be determined by the *class or species* that you're part of rather than some *individual* characteristic? Shouldn't we think of having rights as an individual matter?

MARK: Good point. I'll need to think more about that. I'm sure it'll come up again tomorrow.

MARIA: You bet it will. I'll make sure of it, especially since I'll be reading my paper tomorrow.

MARK: Well, I need to go. Can we pick this up again tonight?

MARIA: Sure.

LARRY: Fine with me.

CAROL: Yes, see you tonight. Same place, same time.

AFTER DINNER

They return to the bar at about eight o'clock and are seated at a corner table. They each have a drink.

5. Rape and Incest

CAROL: Well, what now?

LARRY: Here's something that I don't understand about some pro-lifers. I went to a paper this afternoon read by someone who believed that abortion is wrong even in cases of rape or incest. Talk about outrageous! You don't even allow for an exception where a woman is attacked and made pregnant. You'd force her to go through the further agony of having the child. Recall what you've been saying about fetuses having a right to life. How do fetuses resulting from rapes fit in? Do you think that abortions in such cases are also wrong? If so, why? If not, how do you avoid such a conclusion?

CAROL: Well, I do think that women who become pregnant due to rape shouldn't have abortions. Of course, we shouldn't minimize the traumatic experience that the woman has endured, but why compound the problem by killing the child too? In short, it's not the child's fault how it came to exist. It still has the same right to life as any child or fetus. If the woman does not wish to raise the child, as sometimes happens in other cases anyway, then she can put it up for adoption.

LARRY: Unbelievable! What about the woman's right not to be sexually assaulted in the first place?

CAROL: As I said, the woman's rights were initially violated, but then turning around and violating the right to life of the fetus cannot be justified either. And, again, let's not forget that abortions due to rape are at most two-percent of all cases. I agree that it's an important issue, but let's not ignore the large majority of abortions for the sake of an argument about rape and incest cases.

MARK: Well, I don't go as far as Carol on this point. I disagree with her when it comes to the moral permissibility of abortion in these cases. Even though I'm rather conservative on abortion, I'm a bit more moderate on this type of case.

MARIA: But how can you say that after you've just argued that all fetuses have a right to life because they are potential persons, and so on?

MARK: First of all, even a strong right to life can be overridden in exceptional circumstances. We saw that earlier in cases where a woman's life is at stake. Rape and incest are other rare circumstances where the fetus' right to life can be outweighed by other considerations.

LARRY: But on what grounds can you make such a claim? What makes this case so different?

MARK: As you just said, the woman's rights were violated in the first place. Unlike all other cases where two consenting adults voluntarily engage in intercourse knowing that there is always a chance of pregnancy, in rape cases *the woman did not voluntarily* put herself into that situation. She is not responsible at all for becoming pregnant whereas, in every other case, she is partly responsible and should face the consequences by giving birth to the resulting child.

CAROL: But what difference does that make? Why should "involuntariness" mean so much when it comes to taking a life?

MARK: Well, here's an analogy: Suppose that someone broke into your house and kidnaped you. He took you away and hooked you up to someone, Jones, who needs your blood to stay alive. Only your blood will do the job, so to unplug you from Jones would result in killing him. Suppose your kidnapper said it was only for nine months and it may also involve various other ailments that usually accompany pregnancy. Are you *morally obligated* to remain hooked up to Jones? I don't think so, even though Jones still has a right to life. Of course, if someone *wanted* to stay hooked up to Jones, then that would be fine too. But that would be a supreme act of kindness, which I don't think is morally required. Thus, it would be morally permissible to unplug oneself from Jones. Similarly, it is morally permissible to have an abortion in cases of rape and incest. You see the analogy, right?

LARRY: Sounds good to me, although I still wonder about whether or not you're entitled to make such an exception.

CAROL: Interesting, but I have to challenge your analogy. There are two key disanalogies to real life rape cases. First, in real life the child is still biologically *her* child, whereas Jones is a stranger. Second, in real life the pregnant woman is much more free to do other things than your kidnaped woman. I think that these disanalogies are important in limiting the force of your analogy, Mark.

MARK: Well, I don't see how they are enough to show that my analogy is a bad one. I've shown how in a case where a woman is involuntarily connected to another person, she isn't morally obligated to keep that person alive. The same should hold for abortions in rape cases. It's all very sad and tragic, but I don't think it's morally wrong.

MARIA: But then aren't you also saying that virtually any abortion for very young girls is morally permissible?

MARK: I don't think so. Why?

MARIA: Well, as you know, there is the so-called "age of consent" under which a child cannot legally give consent. It's usually around sixteen, although it varies from State to State. So if a thirteen-year-old girl becomes pregnant by any means, wouldn't it be difficult to say that she acted "voluntarily"?

MARK: I suppose so, although that still seems very different than a rape case where the woman is *forced* to have sex *against her will.* However, in underage cases, especially where a much older man is involved, I'm not sure that an abortion would always be wrong. I'd hope that the family of the girl would be supportive enough and that the situation would still not result in an abortion, but perhaps an abortion would be morally permissible if you really have a case of a girl unable to give voluntary consent.

LARRY: I'm glad we can finally agree on something, Mark.

MARK: As a matter of fact, I'd really like to see older men who get young girls pregnant prosecuted for rape more often.

LARRY: You're right, there should be more of an emphasis on that in our legal system. After all, there are statutory rape laws on the books throughout the country. Part of the problem, though, is that it's always preferable to have the cooperation of the victim and her family, and that doesn't always occur for various reasons. And, in incest cases, there are usually all sorts of other complicated family problems as well.

MARK: Sure, but I'm just saying that it might be a wise course of action to take whenever possible. Maybe it would deter the sexual behavior and help to decrease teenage pregnancy.

MARIA: Perhaps. It can't hurt to try.

CAROL: We can all agree with that. However, in today's sex education oriented society where most young girls engaging in sex know exactly what the potential consequences are, including VD, AIDS, and pregnancy, I'm not sure that we should accept the notion that young pregnant girls are so ignorant and are always acting "involuntarily."

LARRY: But even if we all agreed with you, Mark, wouldn't there be some serious practical problems with allowing *only* such rare cases to be legal? How, for example, do you propose to make sure that a girl was raped before she is allowed to have an abortion?

MARK: Good question. I realize that it would be difficult. I guess we could require that women submit to certain routine physical and psychological tests to determine whether or not they've been raped. As you know, there's usually some clear physical evidence of forced sexual intercourse. We could also require the woman to describe her attacker if possible. And so on. I understand that this might be difficult for the woman, but it could also help us to find rapists and to prosecute them successfully.

LARRY: Perhaps, but aren't you also afraid that other desperate pregnant women will lie about being raped in order to have an abortion?

MARK: That may happen, but hopefully such desperate lies can be clearly distinguished from the real cases. I agree that it could be a difficult practical problem, but it seems worth the effort in order to eliminate the vast majority of abortions that occur every day.

6. Again: Autonomy versus Beneficence

LARRY: I'd like to shift back to the issue of autonomy and self-determination. Remember our discussion yesterday?

MARK: Sure.

LARRY: Well, the principle of autonomy is also very crucial to the abortion debate.

MARIA: Yes. The expression "the right to choose" is often used to emphasize the idea that a woman should have the right to do as she wishes.

CAROL: What did you have in mind, Larry?

LARRY: Basically just that pro-choice advocates believe that the principle of autonomy clearly outweighs the principle of beneficence on this issue. A woman's freedom or liberty shouldn't be restricted in the abortion decision. This is probably the main reason for my pro-choice stand, aside from our earlier discussion about who has a right to life.

CAROL: That's a common way of phrasing the issue. As you know, most conservatives prize individual liberty whether it's a free market economy, freedom of religion, or freedom from burdensome federal regulations. However, abortion is very different. No one should have the right to choose *to kill someone.* Surely that's a legitimate point where one's autonomy should be restricted by the government and the law.

MARK: Exactly. That's why pro-lifers believe that the principle of beneficence outweighs autonomy here. The main reason is the obvious fact that the act of abortion harms someone else; namely, the child. As a matter of fact, the child is not only harmed, but killed. Remember that even the principle of autonomy doesn't say that we can do whatever we want; rather, it says the we ought to be able to do what we want *provided that one's actions do not harm others and/or oneself.* So the principle of beneficence must take priority for the sake of the life of the child. We should protect the life of the unborn. This is very different from voluntary euthanasia cases where at least there is no one *else* being killed as a result of the patient's choice.

LARRY: But what do you mean by 'others' in the expression 'harm others'?

MARK: Well, other human beings, of course.

LARRY: But that's not how I understand the principle of autonomy. It should be taken as: persons ought to be able to do what they wish provided that their actions do not harm other *people* and/or oneself.

CAROL: Are we going to start that again?

LARRY: No, but you can't ignore our earlier discussion in this context. Indeed, it really sheds some light on this point. You think that killing another genetic human being or potential person is virtually always wrong, so beneficence will outweigh autonomy. But we don't agree with that position and, since no person is killed or harmed in an abortion, the woman's autonomy should not be restricted. Autonomy outweighs beneficence.

MARK: Interesting, but I've nothing to add to our earlier discussion. I agree, however, on the importance here of our earlier debate about the moral status of the fetus. *Normally*, of course, there is no question that a right to life outweighs any right to choose. My right to choose does not legally or ethically allow me to kill you.

LARRY: Sure, and that's why the issue so often turns on the status of the fetus; for example, whether it has a right to life at all. If so, why? If not, why not? And that's what we talked about this afternoon.

CAROL: Fine, but there's also growing evidence that having an abortion can be very harmful *to oneself*, which is also mentioned in these two principles. Remember?

LARRY: Yes, but how do you mean?

CAROL: Well, for example, abortions can be destructive to women both physically and psychologically. Almost half of women who have abortions suffer from some kind of physical complication traced to the procedure, such as cuts to the uterus or excessive bleeding. Some women even die from abortion procedures. It's too bad you really don't hear much about them through the mainstream media. They're so biased against pro-lifers, and they do everything they can to keep the pro-choice position from looking bad.

Psychologically and emotionally, many woman who have abortions will later suffer through problems ranging from nightmares and depression to serious guilt over having killed their child. So even for the woman on purely utilitarian grounds, a good case can be made against a woman having an abortion.

LARRY: Maybe, but I'm not sure I believe your claims.

CAROL: I'd be glad to give you some references and to introduce you to some women I know. What's really sad is that pro-lifers are the ones who try to help these women deal with their problems. We've organized support groups for them. The media ignores all this, and most pro-choicers will do anything to make sure that abortion is perceived as "safe." After all, such information would be bad for business.

LARRY: Even if what you say is true, the old alternative of back-alley abortions is worse.

CAROL: I don't think so. Look, I don't want anyone to have an abortion, back-alley or otherwise. It's wrong and dangerous either way. But, statistically, that argument does not stand up. Since abortion became legal in this country, the number of abortions has dramatically increased from estimates of maybe twenty-thousand per year to over one million per year. So even if the odds of any particular woman suffering bad effects from an abortion have dropped, the total number of women who suffer and die from abortions is much greater than ever before. Even just one-third of one million is much greater than twenty-thousand. Woman are worse off today and are in much more danger.

LARRY: I might agree with you if we could verify some of the statistics that you've been throwing around. I'm not sure that I trust your figures.

MARIA: Me either.

CAROL: Well, let's all do some research when we return home.

MARIA: Fine, but the fact remains that it's still the woman's body. Shouldn't she, morally and legally, be able to do what she wants with it?

CAROL: Not *anything* she wants. It's immoral and illegal to use drugs or to engage in prostitution. Where do pro-choicers get the idea that it's ethical for a woman to do whatever she wants with her body? That's just not true. And, again, abortion involves the killing *of someone else*.

MARK: Right. Getting back to the question of "harming the fetus," there are major inconsistencies in the law and in many pro-choicers views on the matter.

MARIA: Such as?

MARK: For example, suppose I took a baseball bat and attacked a pregnant woman by hitting her in the stomach, resulting in the death of the fetus. Would that be wrong?

MARIA: Sure.

MARK: At any stage of pregnancy?

MARIA: I suppose so.

MARK: Why is it wrong?

MARIA: Partly because of the negative effect on the woman.

MARK: *And* because I killed her fetus or child?

MARIA: Sure.

MARK: My point is that you would be horrified if I did such a thing, and I would surely be arrested for my action. It's against the law not only to attack the woman, but also to cause the death of her fetus. Depending on the stage of pregnancy, I could be arrested for anything ranging from assault to homicide.

MARIA: So?

MARK: Well, the legal system and most people's ethical views do make room for the protection of the life of the fetus. In some States, if I killed a pregnant woman during a drunken driving accident, I could even be arrested for double homicide.

MARIA: Yes, but it depends on the age of the fetus.

MARK: But how can it be so wrong *for me* to kill her fetus if it so right *for her* to have her own fetus killed?

MARIA: Well, I see your problem, but you seem to have in mind cases where the woman *wants* to have the child. So the answer to your question is that if the woman wants to have the child, then the law rightly protects her fetus in the ways you describe. But if she does *not* want the child, then the law permits her to have an abortion.

MARK: That seems odd. The moral worth or value of a fetus depends entirely on whether or not the woman wants the child. So if the woman was driving to an abortion clinic, then it wasn't wrong for me to kill the fetus?

MARIA: Maybe not, except for additional harm to the woman. After all, that's not the safest way for a woman to end her pregnancy.

CAROL: I need to jump in here. This really shows the difference between pro-lifers and pro-choicers. You pro-choicers seem to think that the value of a fetus depends on whether or not the woman wants it. Pro-lifers believe that a fetus has **absolute** or **intrinsic** value; that is, a fetus is precious "in itself." The value of a fetus shouldn't change depending on the attitude of the woman. You make it sound like "wanted" and "unwanted" are adjectives describing the child, but the child is the same. *We* are the ones with the problem: there are unwanting people. Unfortunately, the child pays with its life.

MARIA: Well, a fetus can still have some value even if it's not wanted, but generally you are right: a pro-choicer believes that fetal value is **relational** or **extrinsic**; that is, it depends on the attitude of the pregnant woman and perhaps on the other parent as well.

CAROL: But why should a child pay with its life just because its parents don't want it?

MARIA: Let me put it this way: Only the woman is in the best situation to determine fetal value. She is pregnant and only she knows her particular situation. So the decision must be hers.

CAROL: I don't know what else to say.

MARK: Well, I have a second related problem: Do you all agree that it's wrong for a pregnant woman to use drugs and alcohol during pregnancy?

LARRY: Sure, especially in large quantities.

MARK: Aside from the negative affects on the woman, why is it wrong?

LARRY: Well, it can harm the fetus as it develops and then cause all kinds of physical and psychological problems later.

MARK: Right, the fetus would be injured. So it's wrong, say, for a first trimester pregnant woman to drink or use cocaine regularly. Similarly, it would be wrong for a pregnant woman to have a doctor blind her fetus or have an arm removed from her fetus.

LARRY: Of course.

MARK: Will you agree that, according to virtually all ethical and legal systems, injuring someone is not *as wrong* as killing someone?

LARRY: I suppose so. For example, the penalties for murder are greater than the penalties for assault, rape, and so on.

MARK: So if *injuring* the preborn child is wrong, then shouldn't *killing* it be worse? At the least, if injuring the child is wrong, then shouldn't killing it also be wrong? You would have us believe that injuring the early fetus is wrong, but killing it is not wrong at all? I really don't understand such a position.

LARRY: I see your point, but this gets back to what Maria said: Once the woman has made the decision to have the child, then she should do everything she can to keep it healthy and to protect it. So that's why it's wrong for a pregnant woman to injure her developing fetus. However, if she doesn't want the child, then it's morally permissible to have an abortion.

MARIA: And, also, injuring the fetus will lead to significant suffering resulting from the drug use. Injuring the preborn child will negatively affect the child throughout its life as a developing person. From a utilitarian point of view, injuring a fetus by using drugs would clearly be wrong.

MARK: Sure, but killing it wouldn't also be wrong?

MARIA: Not necessarily. For one thing, if the fetus is killed, then there wouldn't be the future suffering endured by the injured fetus.

CAROL: This reminds me of yesterday and our disagreement over the sanctity of life versus the quality of life. The pro-lifer believes that the sanctity of life is more important than the quality of life. They should at least be equally important. In answering Mark's questions, you are making it clear that pro-choicers must admit that only the quality of life counts.

MARIA: How do you mean?

CAROL: Well, you are saying that the very life of the child has less value than the quality of the future child's life. That's why you say that injuring it would be wrong, but killing it wouldn't necessarily be wrong. Your concern is only about the potential suffering of a person due to prenatal injury, but not about the very life of that potential person.

MARK: And it's interesting how you use potentiality here. You two seem to be saying (*pointing to Maria and Larry*) that what makes it wrong to injure a fetus is the potential suffering. Potential suffering matters, but being a potential person doesn't matter?

MARIA: Yes, and I think you're both right in the way that you characterize our disagreement. But the fact remains that in the case of an injured fetus, there will eventually be an actual person who suffers. On the other hand, in the case of an aborted fetus, there will be no one who suffers.

LARRY: Perhaps we are really discovering some of our deeper differences. I guess that's partly what philosophy and argument is all about: uncovering some of the presuppositions in one's arguments and beliefs.

MARK: True, but I'm still surprised at what some of those presuppositions are. I was hoping that I'd change your mind and that you'd eventually give up your position.

LARRY: Sorry to disappoint you, Mark, but it's still good for all of us to keep trying. People do change their minds on such issues. Of course, I'm trying to show you why I think you're wrong too.

Carol and Larry just ask for a glass of water while Mark and Maria order diet sodas. The waitress brings the drinks a few minutes later.

7. Feminism, Oppression, and Other Issues

CAROL: Let me return to the media, since I mentioned them earlier.

MARIA: Sure.

CAROL: It bothers me the way that the media always calls us "anti-abortion" or "anti-choice," instead of "pro-life." It's just another way of attempting to portray us in a negative light. I'd like to hear pro-choice advocates called "pro-abortion" sometimes. That's what they really are.

MARIA: No we're not. I'm not in favor of abortion to the exclusion of having the child. The term 'pro-choice' is accurate because we believe that either option is morally permissible in certain circumstances.

LARRY: And "anti-abortion" or "anti-choice" is just as accurate as "pro-life." You are against abortions and against a woman's right to choose abortions -- aren't you, Carol?

CAROL: Yes, but we'd prefer to be called "pro-life" and, anyway, I still think that many of you are really pro-abortion.

LARRY: Why?

CAROL: Well, for one thing, abortion has sadly become a big industry in this country and there are many people who don't want to see the number of abortions decrease. I really don't think that a significant portion of so-called "pro-choicers" would be just as happy if the number of abortions started to decline. There's a disturbing economic factor in all of this now.

MARIA: Maybe, but speaking for myself, I'd be perfectly happy if the number decreased.

CAROL: Another reason that I think many "pro-choicers" are really "pro-abortion" is that they do everything possible to block even the most modest restrictions to abortion.

LARRY: Such as?

CAROL: Well, they'll fight any attempt at, say, parental consent all the way to the Supreme Court. Women can get an abortion without even talking to her spouse. Also, they'll fight a mere twenty-four hour waiting period. I mean, if abortion is supposed to be such a difficult agonizing decision for a woman, then why don't some people even want her to think it over for a day? The only answer is that pro-abortion forces are afraid that women might change their minds. The same goes for attempts to restrict the free speech of pro-lifers outside abortion clinics. We hand out pamphlets with information about fetal development and abortion alternatives. Again, what's so wrong with at least presenting women with an *informed* choice if you really think that both choices are morally permissible? The only answer can be that you really want them to have the abortion.

LARRY: There may be some people like that, but the reason isn't because we're "pro-abortion," but rather because we don't want women harassed outside the clinics, especially if they've already made up their minds.

MARK: How do you know which women have already made up their minds? What's wrong with presenting the alternative? If she has already made up her mind, then she should ignore us. If she hasn't, then we might save her child. Unfortunately, women don't seem to get much of this information inside the clinics. If both options are morally permissible, then why do pro-choicers get so upset when we try to persuade a woman to have her child?

LARRY: Maybe because they don't think you are really helping the women. You often harass them and some religious fanatics turn violent. As you know, abortion doctors have even been killed by so-called "pro-lifers."

MARK: I know, and it's very embarrassing that some pro-lifers would turn to violence. There are lunatics at the fringe of every movement. Some civil rights protests in the sixties were very violent, but that didn't mean that their views were wrong. Anyway, as you know, the vast majority of pro-lifers are peaceful law-abiding people who just want to save life. We want to help women by encouraging them to keep their child.

CAROL: And I resent you calling us "religious fanatics," Larry. The vast majority of us are simply good peaceful people who are gravely concerned about what is happening in this country.

MARK: I agree, Carol, but I do think that linking the pro-life cause so closely to religion can sometimes hurt it.

CAROL: Why?

MARK: Well, for some of the reasons we talked about the other day concerning God's Command theory. For example, if it's perceived that the main or only reason to oppose abortion is based on religion, then it's so easy for our opponents to reject that argument. For example, others may not share those religious beliefs or argue that we shouldn't base our laws on a single religion's doctrines. That's why we must do better to argue for the pro-life position without relying on religious principles. If we don't, we'll never succeed.

CAROL: I'm not sure about that, and for many of us, religion is our strongest argument against abortion.

MARK: I don't agree. Many people of your same faith, such as Maria, don't even agree with you, Carol.

MARIA: Yes and getting back to "pro-choice" versus "pro-abortion," the fact remains that pro-lifers believe that only one of the two options is morally right, whereas we believe that both options are sometimes morally permissible. We don't agree with China's system of forced abortions in certain circumstances; there's a one child limit in China. Now that's pro-abortion!

CAROL: But some of the same "population control" advocates seem to be at work in this country, and it's the wrong way to go. I agree with you that the China policy is terrible. Much the same happens in India and the result is usually that female fetuses are killed at an alarming rate. Most people there want to have a boy. So they have a sonogram and if it's a girl, the woman almost always has an abortion. It makes you wonder what the proportion of men to women will be in twenty or thirty years.

LARRY: Look, the basic point is that we want women to have the choice. You don't. If you don't want to have an abortion, then don't, but how can you tell another woman not to have an abortion? How can you impose your morality on her?

CAROL: But it's not "my" or "your" morality; it's morality itself. If an action is wrong, then one has every right to try to prevent a person from doing it. You are just assuming that abortion is right, which begs the question. For us, it's no different than telling someone not to rape or murder another person. Imagine if someone said "I personally wouldn't rape a woman, but I don't want to impose my morality on any potential rapists." It's absurd, and sounds like some radical form of relativism.

LARRY: Are you saying that women who have abortions are murderers?

CAROL: I guess I wouldn't call them 'murderers,' but they are doing something wrong. We can understand why they want to have an abortion. We can try not to judge them as people or judge their motives or intentions, but they're still killing a child. And abortion doctors are even worse. I'd be more inclined to call them 'murderers.' They should be punished with jail time.

LARRY: How long?

CAROL: Oh, at least a few years for performing an abortion.

LARRY: You see, this is something I don't understand about pro-lifers. On the one hand, you proclaim that "abortion is murder." On the other hand, most of you suggest that the punishment should be nothing for the woman and minimal for the abortionist. You normally wouldn't recommend release or only a three-year jail term for murder, would you?

CAROL: No.

LARRY: So aren't you implicitly acknowledging that an abortion is not the moral equivalent to murder, even if you believe that they're both wrong?

CAROL: I don't think so. Just because two actions are equally morally wrong, it doesn't follow that the punishment must always be the same. There are many other factors involved; for example, the women are also somewhat victimized and the sad fact that abortion is legal makes it more understandable why people do it. Would you be happier if I said that we should punish all of them for twenty-five years to life?

LARRY: No, but at least you'd be more consistent.

CAROL: Perhaps, but I'm sure that Maria would say something

similar about, say, deer hunters. Even though she believes that they commit murder, I doubt she would recommend jail time or the death penalty.

MARIA: Right. I do think they are murderers, and so is anyone involved in producing meat for human consumption. And anyone who eats meat is indirectly involved in murder. However, given our cultural attitudes toward animals and the fact that most people, unfortunately, don't even think about what is happening, I wouldn't recommend imprisonment.

LARRY: I see.

MARIA: But, getting back to abortion, the other point that we're ignoring here is the history of oppression against women. Most of our institutions have been and continue to be male-dominated. Until the feminist movement, women didn't have the kinds of options and freedoms that we enjoy today, although we still have a long way to go.

MARK: But why should one of those freedoms include having an abortion? Are you trying to get even with us men?

MARIA: No. The right to choose an abortion is one way society tells a woman that we respect her autonomy when it comes to reproduction. Thus, it's an important part of women's liberation from oppression in a male-dominated society, and an essential element of feminism.

CAROL: I couldn't disagree with you more. There are pro-life feminists, such as myself, who believe that the way to free ourselves from oppression is *not* to turn around and oppress another group: the unborn. Pitting women against our offspring is destructive and does nothing to advance our cause.

MARIA: What cause do you mean?

CAROL: I thought that feminism was about equal treatment and also about taking mature responsibility for our own lives with hard work and discipline. Using the right to an abortion as a feminist slogan defeats the original purpose of feminism because women appear too weak to cope with unexpected pregnancies and not responsible enough to take proper precautions. We become helpless victims who can't deal with the consequences of our actions. It's terrible. So don't speak on my behalf about abortion and feminism.

MARIA: Fine, but don't you think that you're overstating it? And the fact remains that having the option of abortion gives us a freedom that we need, especially in a male-dominated society. Men are never faced with the same kind of predicament.

MARK: But don't you think that this abortion strategy has backfired?

MARIA: How do you mean?

MARK: Well, if a pregnant woman claims the right to decide *by herself* whether or not to have a child, then that can only diminish the father's responsibility. It's amazing how the father is rarely mentioned in all of these debates.

LARRY: What do you mean?

MARK: How can we expect men to share in child support or child rearing if they can't share in the very decision as to whether or not there is a child in the first place. Why should I be forced to pay child support if I had no say in whether or not the child was born? In short, abortion encourages male irresponsibility and lack of commitment. Ironically, a man can use pro-choice reasoning in his own mind: "Well, I didn't want the child, the contraceptive failed, having a child will interfere with my career or financial situation, and so on." No wonder more and more men think they're exempted from the responsibilities of fatherhood.

MARIA: I do worry about that aspect of abortion, as a general social policy.

MARK: Don't get me wrong: I'm not advocating male irresponsibility. I'm just saying that I don't see how we can say "the abortion decision is entirely up to the woman" and then, if she decides to have the child, turn around and argue that the man must be financially and otherwise responsible. What if he didn't "want" to have the child for whatever reasons? On the other hand, if abortions are illegal, everyone is encouraged to act responsibly.

LARRY: I see what you mean, but I'm not sure that making abortion illegal is the only way to deal with the social problem of "dead beat dads."

MARK: Maybe not, but as it is now, men can simply pursue their sexual pleasures without thinking much of the consequences of pregnancy. When a women becomes pregnant, many men now say to her "that's your problem." And some men will put pressure on vulnerable women by threatening to break off the relationship if she doesn't have the abortion. What a "choice" that is for a woman! And all of this hurts women; it doesn't help them.

MARIA: I still think that we must ultimately leave the decision up to the woman. After all, there are many circumstances where the woman wants to keep the matter very private. That's one reason why I disagree with pro-lifers who make it sound so simple: just put the child up for adoption! But then the woman couldn't keep it a secret, not to mention going through the process of carrying the child for nine months and the labor itself. And there's no guarantee that the child will be readily adopted.

CAROL: Well, I think that pro-choicers are just afraid that the woman would want to keep the child once she started to realize what she was carrying. But, either way, you can't compare the value of a human life to a few months of "inconvenience."

MARIA: But the thought of putting your own child up for adoption can be very difficult psychologically. If you give birth to a child, it may be very difficult to give it up to someone else.

MARK: So you'd prefer that the woman kill the child earlier in the whole process? How selfish can you get? Kill the fetus now, or else you might really become attached to the child and then adoption would be "psychologically" tough on you! I can't believe it.

MARIA: All I'm saying is that an ethics that is sensitive to women's problems should recognize that abortion may, at least sometimes, be the only acceptable recourse for them.

LARRY: You know, I do think that there are some cases where everyone is better off when an abortion occurs.

CAROL: What? Why?

LARRY: We have a tough enough time taking care of *born* children, not only in the United States but elsewhere. There's poverty and poor living conditions for many people, not to mention child abuse. Some people shouldn't have children in certain circumstances, though I'm not saying that we or the government should force them to have abortions. All I'm saying is that abortion can sometimes lessen the number of those unhappy children.

CAROL: Wow! That sounds pro-*abortion* to me. I agree with you that there are serious social and economic problems, but is abortion the solution to them? And why do you assume that those without money will be "unhappy"? Many of us grew up in less than ideal financial circumstances, but that's no reason to promote or sanction abortion. My mother was one of nine children growing up in relative poverty. On your line of reasoning, abortion may have been better for her or some of my aunts and uncles. What a thought! Even if some children will not live the greatest of lives, is that a reason to kill them before they are born?

LARRY: When you look back at it in that way, it sounds bad. But you can't look at it that way. I'm not talking about already born people.

MARK: I know you're not going to like this, Larry, but sometimes when pro-choicers say things like that, I can't help but think there's a latent racism at work.

LARRY: What? Why? I really resent that.

MARK: I knew you would, but when white people talk about "eliminating some of the poor or disadvantaged in our society through abortion" it sounds like a call to poor "inner city" minorities to start having more abortions. After all, over one-third of the abortions since 1973 have been performed on black babies. When you look at the end result, a racist might be very happy and wish to encourage more of it. Abortion can be used as a subtle and legal form of racism.

CAROL: Especially when pro-choicers fight for the federal funding of abortion, such as through medicaid programs. You know that the end result will be more abortions for low income people.

LARRY: I didn't have any particular group in mind. And, as you know, there are plenty of low income whites and higher income blacks.

MARK: Sure, but by talking about dealing with social problems by eliminating children before they're born, you might be perceived as saying that you wish there weren't those people in the first place. What kind of message does that send?

LARRY: A message of concern over the quality of lives -- actual people's lives!

CAROL: I share your concern, but, once again, your emphasis is always on the quality of life at the expense of life itself. On the other hand, a pro-lifer will say what I said yesterday: the sanctity of life itself must outweigh the quality of life. Even a difficult childhood is better than no childhood!

LARRY: I disagree -- at least in some cases.

MARK: Well, I don't know what more to say except to point out again the danger of the slippery slope. In the case of abortion, it's clear that we've already slid far down the slope. People are having abortions in order to get rid of "abnormal" children. Scientists are now even cloning human embryos.

CAROL: Yes, and even worse, there's so-called "fetal tissue research" where they're now using the tissue of aborted fetuses in experiments supposedly designed to cure diseases. It's all rather grotesque and disturbing. What's next? Are women going to get pregnant on purpose and try to sell their fetus' tissues to laboratories? It just goes to show what happens when we treat a fetus as just a "mass of tissue" instead of as a distinct precious human being.

LARRY: I don't think it's so terrible. Fetal tissue research might eventually really help some people suffering from, say, Alzheimer's disease.

MARIA: How about we stop for today? I think we're all a bit tired, and I need to get some sleep so that I'm mentally prepared to read my paper tomorrow.

CAROL: I'll come to hear your paper.

MARIA: Great. Perhaps tomorrow night we can shift from talking about ethics and *human* animals to the way that we ought to treat other animals.

LARRY: I look forward to it.

MARK: Me too.

They settle the bar bill and return to their respective rooms for the night.

THE FOURTH DAY

ANIMALS

Carol, Larry, Mark and Maria are again at the end of the bar at about eight o'clock with drinks in hand.

1. Introduction

MARK: I think you (*pointing to Maria*) wanted to discuss animals tonight. Although I don't agree with you, Maria, I did enjoy your paper this morning.

CAROL: Me too, especially the discussion of animal consciousness.

LARRY: Same here.

MARIA: Thanks. It's important that we're not only concerned about human animals.

CAROL: I agree to the extent that animals are killed and tortured for all sorts of unnecessary reasons. For example, using animals to test cosmetics and shampoo is rather ridiculous.

MARIA: Sure, but we really should discuss the issue in much greater depth. I think that it's all "unnecessary." Eating meat is wrong. Animal experimentation is wrong. Hunting animals is wrong.

LARRY: I try not to eat too much meat, but I sometimes do. The way that animals are raised for food does often seem morally wrong.

MARK: I don't think eating meat is wrong.

CAROL: Neither do I. And animal experimentation is often essential for some biomedical purposes.

MARIA: As a strong animal rights advocate, I believe in the total abolition of the use of animals in science and the elimination of commercial animal agriculture.

CAROL: That must be a real uphill battle for you. You must realize that you are in a rather small minority.

MARIA: Perhaps, but so what? We can slowly start to change things in the right direction and, don't forget, the majority is not always ethically right. I realize there are others in the animal rights movement who don't go as far as I do on this issue, but something is better than nothing.

I mean, tens of millions of animals are used just for experimentation each year, and that's only in the United States. And the kinds of animals range from rabbits, hamsters, dogs, and cats to chimpanzees and apes. The current law allows for it even though some minor changes have been made to ease the suffering of animals, such as in The Animal Welfare Act of 1970. But the conditions in general, such as lack of exercise, isolation, and tiny cages, are very stressful. Animals are still treated as mere property without any rights, and some experiments are absurd.

MARK: Such as?

MARIA: Well, for example, they subject monkeys to radiation which induces vomiting, they smash animals' heads against walls to study head trauma, they do electric shock studies on dogs and primates to study heart rate and blood pressure, and so on. It's terrible.

LARRY: Sure, but you'd be opposed to animal experimentation even if all the suffering were eliminated. Right?

MARIA: Yes, but there's little evidence to suggest that experimenters are willing to change with regard to easing suffering. And most experiments necessarily cause great suffering.

2. Consciousness, Inherent Value, and the Right to Life

MARK: So what's your main reason for opposing animal experimentation?

MARIA: Would you agree that any creature with a right to life shouldn't be used for medical experimentation?

MARK: Yes, if you mean 'used against their will.'

MARIA: Sure, but that's always the case with using animals. They don't ask for animal volunteers!

MARK: Of course.

MARIA: Remember what I said yesterday about consciousness as the key to a right to life?

MARK: Yes. You seemed to have in mind *any* form of consciousness.

MARIA: Right, because consciousness obviously comes in degrees. Humans are capable of having some conscious mental states that many other animals aren't. For example, we can have thoughts about advanced mathematics and philosophical issues whereas dogs can't. There are increasing levels of mental ability up through the evolutionary chain. But the key should be **sentience**; that is, the capacity to suffer and/or experience pleasure. That's the only defensible and non-arbitrary boundary between those organisms that have inherent value and those things that don't.

MARK: I'm not so sure about that. As you know from yesterday, all of us disagree with you. Carol and I think that actual or potential persons, or any member of a species that typically contains persons, have a right to life. So mere consciousness is neither necessary nor sufficient for having a right to life. And Larry thinks that only actual persons have a right to life, so animals do not have a right to life unless they are also considered "persons."

MARIA: Sure, but all of you had to deal with some serious objections. Remember? Infants, mentally defective humans, and so on? Anyway, the reason why consciousness is so important is that any conscious creature, no matter how primitive, will have some sort of desire to continue to live. It should take a very good reason to end such a life, and I don't think that any of the usual reasons given are very strong.

MARK: Well, we can all agree that many animals are conscious creatures all the way down at least to mice, rats, reptiles, and birds. And you're also right about degrees of consciousness. I wouldn't dispute that the animals used in experiments are sentient creatures. It's fairly obvious given their behavior and our knowledge of their brain structure.

MARIA: Good. So then here's the argument from my paper this morning. What's wrong with it?

Maria puts a copy of the argument on the bar. It was a sheet of paper from her morning presentation.

(1) All conscious creatures have inherent value.
(2) All who have inherent value have it equally.
Therefore, (3) All conscious creatures, whether human or not, have equal inherent value.
(4) All who have equal inherent value have an equal right to life.
Therefore, (5) All conscious creatures, whether human or not, have an equal right to life.

And since you agreed that all creatures with a right to life, including humans, shouldn't be used for experimentation, then we shouldn't experiment on any conscious animal!

LARRY: Interesting; it does seem to be logically valid, but are all of the premises true?

MARIA: I think so. I've just explained the rationale behind premise 1. And premise 2 is the only way to ensure nonarbitrariness. For example, if we believe that an infant or a retarded child has the same right to life as you or I, then we should accept premises 1 and 2. Premise 4 is simply the transition from inherent value to a right to life.

LARRY: Well, even if we accept premise 1, the real resistance will be to premises 2 and 4. Even if one agrees with you that all conscious creatures have inherent value, it's not clear that we all have it *equally*, not to mention the transition to an *equal* right to life.

CAROL: Exactly, Larry. And I'd also point out that Maria's view leaves out fetuses.

MARIA: Yes, but only early fetuses before sentience begins. Remember?

CAROL: Sure, but the fact remains that you think any animal with actual consciousness, no matter how primitive, has more value than an early human fetus. Right?

MARIA: Yes, because I don't agree with you on the importance of potentiality. And why do you get so upset by the killing of a one-inch utterly unconscious embryo, and not by the killing or torturing of, say, a clearly conscious cat?

CAROL: Well, because a potential human *person* is far more valuable than an actual cat. (*Maria is shaking her head.*)

MARK: I agree. Indeed, only the potential person, not the cat, has a right to life. Of course, that doesn't mean we should kill and torture cats unnecessarily. I'm sure that a lot could be done to reduce animal suffering.

LARRY: As you know, I think that neither the cat nor the early fetus has a right to life. Neither are actual persons, but go on, Maria.

MARIA: Anyway, one way to put my point is that there shouldn't be any animal experimentation for the same reasons that it's wrong to use infants or mentally defective humans. Here's the test: an experiment on an animal is justifiable only if it's so important that the use of mentally defective humans would also be justifiable. I assume you'd oppose those experiments.

CAROL: Of course.

MARK: Of course.

LARRY: I guess so.

MARIA: Good. Well, then, that would effectively eliminate animal experimentation. It's hard to imagine an experiment that would be so important.

LARRY: Maybe, but why is that the test?

MARIA: Because all conscious creatures have equal inherent value. And, as a matter of fact, many animals used in experiments, such as apes and monkeys, have superior psychological capacities to mentally defective humans.

CAROL: Perhaps, but mentally defective humans are still humans!

MARIA: So? They're all conscious and don't want to suffer. They all want to continue to live. That's what counts.

CAROL: I don't agree.

MARIA: Why?

CAROL: As I see it, there are *three* major arguments in favor of animal experimentation: one based on religion, a second based on the simple fact that we're humans and animals aren't, and a third having to do with some of the psychological differences you've already raised.

MARIA: Those are the three main alleged justifications for animal experimentation, but none of them stand up to close scrutiny. Let's discuss them one at a time, as best we can.

3. Religion and Animals

CAROL: Okay. First, only humans have immortal souls and, in that sense, we are very special in God's eyes.

MARIA: I believe in God too, but I don't see how you could rest your position on a controversial metaphysical belief. Why make such an assumption in order to defend animal experimentation?

LARRY: I have to agree with Maria here.

CAROL: But it's clear from the Bible that the Judeo-Christian God created animals ultimately to serve the purposes of humans. God gave us "dominion over" animals, and so animals don't have moral standing. Animals are here for our use. To put it in Kant's language, only *rational* animals should be treated as ends in themselves. So lower animals only have *instrumental value*; that is, value as a means to human ends. That's what Kant believed.

MARIA: Well, that's a distorted interpretation of the concept of "God's dominion."

CAROL: Why?

MARIA: I think it means that we have an important responsibility to animals in the sense of a proper stewardship of God's creation. And so God wants us to be responsible in our treatment of animals.

MARK: And, again, remember the problems with God's Command theory of ethics? You have the same problems here, Carol.

CAROL: Maybe, but why does "being responsible" entail *the abolition* of animal experimentation or becoming a vegetarian? I agree that we could be more responsible in our treatment of animals, but I don't see how we are led to Maria's conclusions.

MARIA: You're not led to my position for that reason alone, but I've already given other reasons in support of it. At this point, I'm simply replying to your religion-based argument in favor of animal experimentation.

CAROL: Fine, but there's a long history of animal sacrifice and of eating meat in the religious tradition, also mentioned in various classical Biblical passages. Anyone who reads those passages, for example in Genesis, can clearly see that no conservative Christian can be a vegetarian on religious grounds. Maybe this shouldn't be the main reason for a pro-experimentation view, but it's at least one reason.

MARIA: But there are also New Testament passages where the people only eat fish, nuts, and vegetables.

LARRY: And let's not forget that the Bible has been used to support the unequal treatment of races and of women, and those views are now widely rejected. Why should it be any different for the portrayal of animals in the Bible? I love the way that Christians pick and choose what to take literally in the Bible.

CAROL: Well, just because some groups or individuals distort a document to make it support their views doesn't mean that we should attribute their perspective to the document itself. Inequality of men and women in terms of their proper roles and responsibilities is, of course, taught in the Bible, but sexism and racism, as you seem to have in mind, is certainly not a Biblical teaching.

MARK: But why should we take the Biblical portrayal of animals as literally supporting some moral position?

CAROL: Well, again, at the least, because humans have souls. That's one big difference between us and animals, which is not open to interpretation.

MARIA: Maybe, but some religious philosophers have often spoken of the "animal soul" in addition to the "rational human soul." However, I can see pursuing this line of argument with you, Carol, would be a waste of time.

CAROL: Probably. Look -- leaving religion aside, the fact remains that we're humans and they're animals. That's enough justification for animal experimentation by itself.

4. Speciesism

MARIA: Well, that's simply unjustifiable speciesism.

CAROL: What?

MARIA: **Speciesism** is a prejudice or attitude of bias in favor of the interests of members of one's own species and against those of the members of other species. It's the devaluing of animals *just because* they are animals. As far as I'm concerned, it's the moral equivalent to racism and sexism. It's treating others as inferior based purely on biological factors and mere appearances.

CAROL: That's an absurd analogy.

MARIA: Why? You said something similar about fetuses yesterday. Why not agree that the oppression of animals should also be eliminated? Merely being of a different species cannot morally justify such radical differences in treatment.

CAROL: I don't see how you can compare racism and sexism to so-called 'speciesism.' As a matter of fact, even just calling it 'speciesism' and making your analogy is insulting to women and minorities. You're comparing women to pigs and cats. How absurd! But I guess you really do believe that we all have equal value.

MARIA: Yes, especially when it comes to *equal treatment* in cases of painful experimentation.

MARK: Maybe using the term 'speciesism' is a good strategy. After all, no one wants to be accused of bigotry or racism. Maybe we should start calling pro-choice abortion advocates 'fetusists' who practice 'fetusism.'

MARIA: Very funny.

MARK: Well, seriously, I really don't see how you can compare speciesism with racism and sexism.

MARIA: I've just explained it. Let me try it another way: Suppose that some vastly stronger and more intelligent creatures from outer space invaded Earth. They live here for a while, and then they decide to capture some of us and use us in experiments. Would they be morally justified in doing so?

CAROL: Of course not.

MARIA: But I don't see how a speciesist supporter of animal experimentation can consistently argue that the superior aliens are morally wrong. On the other hand, I can explain why they are wrong: all of us are sentient creatures. And speciesiem is wrong.

CAROL: Why can't we also conclude that they're wrong?

MARIA: Because their reasoning would be the same as yours regarding other animals. We can imagine one of their scientists explaining to us how they are so much more intelligent than us, and they would do their best to minimize our pain and keep us in clean cages. They might even "regret" having to perform painful experiments on us, but it's "necessary" for the benefit of their own species. Perhaps they even enjoy our company or are amused by us. Maybe they even keep some of us as pets, but, in the end, we are only "human."

CAROL: That's an interesting science fiction story, but it's difficult to know what to make of it.

MARIA: Well, use your imagination, would they be morally justified or not?

CAROL: Of course not.

MARIA: But why? They are using the same speciesist reasoning that you did earlier. Maybe they even observed how we treat animals, and then came to believe that they should do the same to us.

CAROL: But the fact remains that we have immortal souls and are made in God's image. And, also, we're people and animals aren't.

MARIA: Let's not get back into that.

CAROL: Well, what more can I say?

LARRY: Maybe Maria is right and we'd just have to face the fact that the aliens would be morally justified in experimenting on us, as long as we continue to treat animals the way we do. It's a frightening thought, but we can just hope that such a scenario doesn't occur and be glad that we're on top of the evolutionary chain on Earth.

MARIA: I'm glad you mentioned evolution. Although I do believe that *the universe* was created by God, I also believe in evolution. It seems to me that speciesism is inconsistent with the main lesson of evolution; namely, the message of evolutionary kinship between humans and animals. The time has come for us to extend our ethics to include a concern for animal suffering. We're all animals that come from common ancestors.

CAROL: I don't believe in evolution, but I guess we don't want to discuss the merits of evolutionary *theory* at this point.

MARK: Please no, but I don't see how any scientifically informed person could reject evolution; the fossil record and the scientific evidence is there. But getting back to your point, Maria, it seems to me that you conveniently ignore another very important principle of evolution.

MARIA: What?

MARK: Probably the phrase that is most commonly associated with Darwin: survival of the fittest. I mean, if you're going to use evolution to support your position, then I think you're in trouble.

MARIA: Exactly how?

MARK: Well, look at how animals treat each other in order to survive. They eat each other and, if they were smart enough, I'm sure they'd experiment on each other in order to ensure the survival of their species. Evolution tells us that survival is the most primitive biologically-based cause of much of animal behavior. The forces of natural selection have shaped all animals in such a way that we want to maximize the chances of the survival of our genes and our species.

MARIA: Maybe, but why can't we rise above that behavior when it's not necessary to act that way toward our fellow creatures?

MARK: Maybe we can be "above it" when it's not necessary for the survival of our species, but most experimentation is necessary for our survival. It's at least necessary for minimizing our suffering and increasing the quality of our lives. It's a way of ensuring the survival of our species. Also, Maria, you seem to want to have it both ways: on the one hand, we're just animals with animal ancestors and we should all be treated equally; on the other hand, we're so superior to animals that we should refrain from acting in the way that they act or would act in similar situations.

MARIA: Well, I don't deny that normal human beings are superior intellectually to animals, although I do wonder about some people. And I also believe that only we have some ability to control our behavior. Perhaps only we have free will. But, again, the main point has to do with suffering and sentience. That's what we share with animals and that's what should count.

MARK: But, from an evolutionary point of view, isn't it somewhat natural to want to take care of one's own? For example, a mother has a special duty toward her child even if it's at the expense of another's child. Suppose that she could only save one in a house fire: either her child or the neighbors child. No one would fault her for saving her own.

MARIA: Probably not, but I'm not sure how this supports speciesism. I might save one of my dogs over some human stranger, and I don't think that I should be faulted for that either. After all, my dogs are very much part of "my family." This shows that it's not merely one's species as such, but it's also who one cares about or loves. It may be "natural" to save one's own, but that won't support speciesism or animal experimentation.

MARK: But would you save one of your dogs over one of *your* children?

MARIA: I guess not.

MARK: Would you save an animal "stranger" over a human stranger?

MARIA: Probably not.

MARK: So if the speciesist claim is that "under some circumstances we should give greater weight to our species over another species," then survival of the fittest and our natural tendency to endure as a race *would* support animal experimentation. Just as a mother has a special duty to her own child, so we owe a special duty to members of our own species.

MARIA: But you make it sound as if *either* we continue to experiment on animals *or* we will be severely negatively affected as a species. That's clearly a false dilemma. For one thing, most experiments don't result in any important medical knowledge. Your analogy to the difficult moral choice faced by the mother is a poor one. There's no current animal experiment where if we don't perform it, we will die. I mean, it's not as if we either experiment on animals or we die.

MARK: I'm not so sure about that, and surely many *past* experiments have saved human lives and decreased human suffering dramatically. So even if no human *now* would die or suffer greatly if we eliminated all current experiments, it's very likely that many future people would.

LARRY: I agree with Mark here. Just think of the polio vaccine and all kinds of pills and medications. Many mammals, including monkeys, were used to gain such medical knowledge.

MARIA: I don't deny that some benefits have been gained from animal experimentation. And maybe I'm hypocritical to the extent that I sometimes use such medication, but ---

LARRY: That's interesting. I assume you had your children immunized, and that you'd use medication if, say, you developed a heart problem.

MARIA: Yes, but my point is that just because some benefits are gained, it doesn't follow that the experimentation is morally right. It's no different than if we did the same to human beings and then gained some medical knowledge. It might be difficult to resist using the results of those experiments, but that doesn't mean the experiments were right in the first place or that we should continue to perform them.

LARRY: I don't agree. Perhaps it all comes back to the moral status of animals, in terms of their rights. If you don't believe that animals have a right to life, then the only issue becomes a purely utilitarian one; that is, the balance of animal suffering against human pleasure or the lowering of human suffering.

CAROL: Right, and a strong case can be made that the good outweighs the bad. Again, think of all the medications we have. And, of course, we shouldn't forget that the law requires us to test drugs very carefully before they're used on humans. Just imagine the benefits of a cure for AIDS or cancer!

MARIA: I'm not so sure that the good outweighs the bad, even if you insist on phrasing it in such crude utilitarian terms. Moreover, we rarely *know* what will result from animal experimentation. There's so much trial and error and absurd duplication of experiments. It's easy to look back and claim success, but it's not that simple.

CAROL: But you seem to be saying that *if* it did come down to a choice between my child dying and experimenting on an animal, you'd let my child die. I can't accept that.

MARIA: I have nothing more to add.

The bartender stops by and takes their order for more drinks. The drinks are placed on the bar within a minute.

5. Psychological Differences

LARRY: Well, I still think that psychological factors are the most important way to justify animal experimentation. For example, I'd argue that experiments on animals are morally permissible partly because they are not persons. That is, they don't have certain psychological capacities, such as an ability to reason or self-consciousness.

MARIA: But, first of all, I again don't see how lacking those psychological capacities can justify experimentation. The question shouldn't be "Can they reason?" but rather "Can they suffer?" Perhaps some insects, worms, snails, and small fish are not conscious at all, given their lack of requisite brain structure. However, it's clear that all animals used in experiments or for food are capable of suffering. I mean, who could deny that such animals have conscious mental states when we often attribute to them rather complex conscious visual and auditory experiences?

Second, animals don't entirely lack the psychological capacities of reason and self-consciousness.

LARRY: What do you mean?

MARIA: Well, self-consciousness and rationality come in degrees. Depending on what we mean by 'self-consciousness' and 'reason,' most animals probably do have such abilities to some extent. For example, self-consciousness ranges from a primitive awareness of one's own pains and feelings to more sophisticated acts of deliberation. Surely virtually all animals are at least capable of the former, and there's some evidence to suggest that higher mammals even deliberate to some extent. They show evidence of "figuring out" what to do in various challenging or unexpected situations, both in experimental and natural environments. These abilities not only seem to require self-consciousness, but also some form of reasoning capacity. Again, 'reasoning' could mean anything from the "ability to make simple inferences or the ability to solve simple problems" to the more sophisticated "capacity to think abstractly about theoretical physics, mathematics, philosophy, logic, ethics, and so on."

LARRY: I see. I guess I don't question that most animals are self-conscious or can reason *to some extent*, although I'd need to know more in order to judge how far down the evolutionary scale it goes.

MARK: I basically agree with Maria on the psychological capacities of animals, although I'm not convinced that any reasoning occurs in some lower animals, such as mice, squirrels, and so on. However, apes and monkeys clearly can reason to some extent.

MARIA: This is a whole other major issue of interest to psychologists and ethologists. But my point here is only that even if you require self-consciousness and reasoning for a right to life and personhood, many animals would still qualify as long as you allow for degrees of those psychological capacities.

LARRY: But even if you're right that personhood, self-consciousness, and reasoning ability comes in degrees, wouldn't it then make more sense to hold that there are corresponding degrees of rights-to-life or, as you mentioned earlier, "inherent value"?

MARIA: How so?

LARRY: Well, I find it hard to believe, as you seem to, that there are only two categories: those things that have the same inherent value and the same moral rights that we do, and those that have none at all, such as rocks and trees. You don't allow for degrees of value or moral rights in the same way that you allow for degrees of psychological capacities.

MARK: Right, Larry. Why must all conscious creatures have *equal* inherent value? Why must all creatures with inherent value have an *equal* right to life? Given the enormous psychological differences between us and animals, it's difficult for me to believe that we have the same right to life as a frog. And that's assuming that frogs have a right to life in the first place.

MARIA: I'm glad we've come back to my original argument.

LARRY: Fine, but why is inherent value an all-or-nothing matter?

MARIA: As I said earlier, because sentience is all-or-nothing. Either an animal suffers pain or it doesn't. The degrees of self-consciousness and rationality are important psychological differences between species, but sentience is that which unites us. Also, all conscious animals have some capacity for memory and for anticipating the future. It's clear that animals want to continue to live, and so we shouldn't end their lives.

LARRY: It still seems that a more plausible alternative to your view would be that animals don't have rights, but we are obligated not to be cruel to them.

CAROL: Haven't we overlooked another difference between animals and humans?

MARIA: What?

CAROL: It's related to our psychological differences, but it's a key *moral* difference. Humans are uniquely self-legislative and morally autonomous; that is, only humans lay down moral laws for ourselves in a society. Animals lack this capacity for free moral judgment. We're able to act on moral judgments, whereas animals aren't. This isn't to say that we always act morally, but only that we're capable of acting on the basis of moral judgments. On the other hand, animals don't deliberate over what is right or wrong and then act accordingly. Only we have this ability, which seems crucial to having rights at all.

MARIA: Why?

CAROL: Well, because a "right" is a claim or potential claim that one might exercise against another. So being able to comprehend and act on moral laws is essential to having rights.

MARIA: Again, I don't see why having these sophisticated psychological abilities is necessary for having a right to life. And the real problem for those who believe that animals lack rights due to their lower psychological capacities is the one I mentioned earlier: Infants and mentally defective human beings would also not have a right to life if abstract reasoning, advanced self-consciousness, and the capacity for free moral judgment were required. Also, there will always be animals that have greater psychological abilities than some individual humans. So how can you argue that a newborn infant or a mentally defective human has a right to life and that a monkey or a dog does not?

CAROL: I agree that this is a serious problem, but only if you base our position solely on psychological differences. I still think that religious and speciesist replies can be made here.

LARRY: As I said yesterday, I don't even think that newborn infants and mentally defective humans have a right to life. However, as with animals, that doesn't mean we should do anything we want to them, such as making them suffer unnecessarily.

MARK: Well, I don't accept Larry's answer to your problem, Maria, partly for the reasons we discussed yesterday. Also, you (*pointing to Larry*) do seem to think that there's something wrong with experimenting on newborns generally, whereas you've yet to say that about animals.

LARRY: I guess so. Perhaps some speciesism is also at work in my position.

MARK: But, anyway, to answer Maria's problem, we could again respond with the notion of 'potentiality.' Even though newborn humans don't have advanced reasoning abilities or have any sense of morality, they will develop these characteristics over time. And, as we saw yesterday, the same goes for fetuses. On the other hand, a cat or an elephant has no such potential. That's why normal fetuses and infants must belong to the moral community and why cats don't.

MARIA: But what about mentally defective humans?

MARK: Well, the same kind of logic applies although, unlike normal infants, defective humans will not *naturally* develop those capacities. We can still say, however, that they have the *faculty* of reason, but simply can't use it well or at all. The idea is that we could ideally correct their condition so that their full intellectual capacities could be manifested. Animals, on the other hand, can't be made to have the capacity in the first place. We can't "cure" a cat and give it advanced reasoning abilities. We can't prevent a cat from being a cat! That's its nature.

MARIA: Interesting, but your explanation sounds a bit unrealistic and unnecessarily complex. And, of course, in order to find the cures you're talking about, scientists will no doubt kill and torture millions of animals.

CAROL: But the point is similar to one we made yesterday about an essential feature of human beings as opposed to animals. It's a fairly straightforward way to determine which creatures have a right to life: If members of your species *generally* or *typically* have the features of personhood, then you have a right to live whether or not you individually possess all those features. So humans who are unable, because of some disability, to reason abstractly or to solve complex problems aren't therefore left out.

MARIA: But why shouldn't we treat animals *individually* for the purposes of ethics? Why should having a right to life depend on what is "typical" in a species? Why do we need to know what *kind* of animal it is before we decide whether or not we should experiment on it? There is the danger of determining what is ethical in terms of one's "class" rather than by one's individual make-up. If an individual ape or dog right now has greater psychological capacities than a mentally defective human right now, why is it ethical to experiment on the animal and wrong to experiment on the human?

MARK: I thought I already explained why. And perhaps there is also some speciesism involved as well.

MARIA: But shouldn't we think of rights as an individual matter to be determined by individual characteristics?

MARK: I don't think so. The individual *has the rights*, but *why it has the rights* partly depends on the kind of thing it is; that is, the class of organism that it belongs to. If being a person is generally characteristic of your species, then all members of that species have a right to life. This protects the abnormal, the defective, and the unborn from being killed. That's the way it should be. If we rely solely on individual psychological characteristics, then we may end up with the problems that Larry faced yesterday.

MARIA: But that's only because you and Larry are using such sophisticated psychological capacities. In contrast, using sentience as the criterion would cover the same individuals.

MARK: Except for pre-conscious fetuses, right?

MARIA: Right. Of course someone might be pro-animal-rights *and* pro-life on abortion, but I'm not.

MARK: Me either, but it's certainly another possible position.

LARRY: Getting back to psychological differences, here's another way to think about it from a legal point of view. An act can be criminal only when there's a guilty mind involved. This is related to the capacity for making moral judgments, and to forming the requisite motive and intent. This is why a person or the government can bring charges against someone for violating one's rights. However, animals can't commit crimes, and so animals shouldn't be included in the moral community.

MARK: Right, what are we supposed to do when a dog or a bear attacks a human being? Maybe we should arrest the animal and put it in handcuffs, two pair, and ---

MARIA: Very funny, but even if no animal can commit a crime, why can't we still extend to animals the same respect for life that we extend to newborn infants and to defective humans?

LARRY: Because animals cannot and could never return that same respect.

MARK: Right, the fact remains that animals are very different than humans in many ways, and so we can't treat them the way we treat each other.

MARIA: But I didn't say that we had to treat animals *the same in every way*. That would be absurd and not very practical. All I'm saying is that we should treat them the same in one very basic way: don't torture or kill them for experimental purposes.

6. Reduction and Substitution

MARK: I agree with you to the extent that the number of animals used in experimentation could be greatly reduced.

MARIA: I guess that's better than nothing.

CAROL: One thing that could be done is to reduce the duplication of experiments when they aren't absolutely necessary for validating the original research.

MARIA: We try to encourage that, but we run into the problem that many scientists around the country don't share information the way you might think. There's limited coordination between different laboratories, partly because they each want to be the first to discover some new cure or drug. So competition often breeds an atmosphere of limited cooperation.

LARRY: And I'm sure they each must justify the federal grant money they receive for their research.

MARIA: Yes, so it's a difficult battle.

MARK: The only point in their defense, I think, is that federal regulations rightly require the testing of new drugs on animals before we're exposed to them. I guess we wouldn't want it any other way. I certainly don't see how we could abolish animal research and continue advances in medicine. Sooner or later, a drug must be tried on a living animal.

MARIA: Maybe, but another possibility is to use computer technology more frequently.

CAROL: How?

MARIA: Well, they can input information into a computer containing a three-dimensional image of an animal that mimics its biological functions. The computer provides an output based on all the information. This can be done hundreds of times without killing or injuring a single animal.

CAROL: But eventually live animals must be used.

MARIA: Not necessarily, but even if so, at least millions of animals will be spared every year. And many pointless and wasteful experiments might be recognized as such long before live animals are used. The technology in this area is amazing, but it's underused and not financed to the extent that it should be.

MARK: Interesting. I'd also like to see more substitution of higher animals with lower animals. I know you think it's all wrong, Maria, but to many of us there is something very different about, say, using a rat instead of a monkey.

LARRY: Yes, perhaps due to the degrees of self-consciousness and rationality that we discussed earlier.

CAROL: Well, there is one major problem with that: scientists will tend to want animals that are biologically closer to us in order to get more scientifically valid results. There is the tension between wanting to use higher animals for that reason and yet, also, trying to substitute lower animals whenever possible.

MARK: Sure but, whenever possible, they should try to use lower instead of higher animals.

MARIA: Unfortunately, they really don't. Tens of thousands of primates are used every year, not to mention dogs and cats.

LARRY: Maybe they could do a better job of controlling the pain in experiments by using more anesthetics and tranquilizers. If the pain and unnecessary suffering is mainly what's objectionable, then why don't they do more along these lines?

MARIA: Well, it's not only the pain from the experiments themselves, but also from the living conditions. And it seems to me that most experiments *necessarily* cause pain and suffering. It's almost impossible to have one without much of the other.

MARK: Also, I'm sure that scientists will tell you that using anesthetics and tranquilizers would negatively affect their results. I mean, pain killers would distort an experimental result in a way that would defeat the purpose of the experiment. The tests need to be controlled without combining different drugs. Otherwise, the results wouldn't be reliable.

LARRY: I see.

MARIA: Excuses, excuses!

CAROL: Maybe they could also use fewer animals for teaching

purposes in colleges and medical schools. Perhaps it's sometimes necessary to have medical students actually use animals, but it's not always necessary. At least sometimes, a teacher using a single animal for demonstration would be good enough. This could be done much more often.

MARIA: As I said before, it's better than nothing. At least we can agree on that much.

7. Vegetarianism

LARRY: Maria, let me ask you this question: do you think that if you believe animal experimentation is wrong, then you must also believe that eating meat is wrong?

MARIA: Sure. At least it's possible for those who support animal experimentation to argue that it's somehow necessary for our survival or for our health, although I still think that's wrong. However, there can be no such argument for eating meat.

LARRY: I agree that *if* one opposes animal experimentation, then one should also think that eating meat is morally wrong. However, I don't think that the opposite is true for the reason you just gave.

MARIA: But what do you think of eating meat?

LARRY: I mentioned before that I try not to eat meat, including chicken and fish, but sometimes I do. I guess I do think it's sometimes wrong, but only because of the way that the animals are treated. If animals could be raised and killed painlessly for food, then eating meat would be morally permissible. So, at most, I'm what we might call a **conditional vegetarian**; that is, one who believes that the wrongness of using animals for food depends on whether our treatment of them causes great suffering.

MARIA: I see. Well, as you know then, I'd be an **unconditional vegetarian**; that is, someone who believes that it's always wrong to eat meat regardless of how they are raised or are killed. This should be clear from what I've said so far. Causing suffering is wrong, but killing an animal for food is also wrong no matter how it's done. It's wrong to kill anything that wants to live, even if it is done painlessly. It was difficult for me to watch all of you eating meat at lunch yesterday, but I didn't want to say anything at that time.

LARRY: I understand your position, but do you eat any egg or dairy products?

MARIA: I'm a **lacto vegetarian**. So I also don't eat any egg products, but I do eat dairy products such as cheese and milk. There are other possibilities. For example, **ovo vegetarians** eat egg products but abstain from dairy products, whereas **lacto-ovo vegetarians** eat both eggs and dairy products. And **vegans** won't eat any animal products whatsoever. There are other categories as well, but the common feature is that we don't eat any meat and that includes chicken and fish.

CAROL: Are you able to get proper nutrition in your diet? I mean, if you don't get enough vitamins and iron in your diet, then isn't that a good health reason to eat meat?

MARIA: It's really no problem at all. There are vegetables, beans, fruits, and so on. And, as a lacto vegetarian, I also get the nutritional benefits of cheeses and milk related products. And, of course, there are always vitamin supplements if one has any doubts. Even vegans do just fine. If anything, being a vegetarian can benefit one's overall health rather than damage it. As you know, many health problems are associated with eating meat, especially in the quantities that most Americans consume.

CAROL: So it's not necessary to eat meat for health reasons?

MARIA: Absolutely not.

CAROL: Then I guess it would be difficult to make the analogy to experimentation by arguing that eating meat is also necessary for our health and survival.

MARIA: Right, especially now.

MARK: What do you mean by 'especially now'?

MARIA: Well, perhaps years and years ago when there was limited knowledge of these matters and killing animals for food was almost a matter of survival, I could understand why it was done. Perhaps it wasn't even wrong.

MARK: Why?

MARIA: Because it may really have been analogous to self-defense and pure survival. But that's not true now.

MARK: So it wasn't wrong to kill and eat animals centuries ago, but it is now? I'm not sure I understand that view. It almost sounds like a kind of relativism.

MARIA: Not necessarily. It's just that knowledge and technology has progressed to the point that eating meat is no longer 'necessary' in any sense of the term. And if eating meat *was* morally permissible *only because* it was a necessary source of food and nutrition, then it's clearly no longer morally permissible today.

MARK: But part of the technology we've developed involves such inventions as electric freezers. So instead of hunting our food for pure survival like our ancestors did, we've used our intelligence to raise, kill, and store animals on a mass scale. So why is that wrong now?

MARIA: Again, because it's not necessary now.

MARK: But our intelligence is part of what we've used to survive. Remember our discussion on speciesism and survival of the fittest? I mean, eating meat now and raising animals the way we do is just a natural extension of the way we did it in the past.

MARIA: So just because we always did it, it's right to do now?

MARK: In this case, yes. I don't see why the changes in technology and knowledge should suddenly make eating meat wrong. That's not how we usually reason about these ethical issues. Unless you are a relativist, you'd say that slavery was always wrong regardless of the surrounding circumstances. So if killing animals for food is wrong, it was always wrong. The act itself was wrong. It sounds odd to say that it might have been right in the past, but not in the present.

MARIA: But there's no current reason for us to have to eat meat.

MARK: I don't understand. Getting back to survival of the fittest, is it wrong for a cat to kill a mouse? Is it wrong for a lion to eat a zebra? Was it wrong for the T Rex to eat a Brontosaurus? Do animals have the right not to be eaten by other animals?

MARIA: No, but those cases are different.

MARK: Why? I mean, animals eat each other all the time, they always have, and they always will. You make it sound like animals live in some beautiful happy harmony together. How absurd! Maybe you should watch more of those PBS nature shows.

MARIA: Funny, but I'm well aware of animal eating habits. And, anyway, it's just not true that *all* animals eat each other, if that's what you meant. As a matter of fact, the animals that most people eat don't eat meat at all; for example, pigs, lambs, and cows are vegetarians!

MARK: Good point, but how can it be right for *some* animal to kill a cow and eat it, and yet wrong if we do it? Isn't that an odd consequence of your view?

MARIA: No. When animals do it, they don't know any better and can't help they're instinctive behavior. However, we can do otherwise. We don't have to eat animals and we can use our ability to reason to develop alternatives.

MARK: But, again, Maria, you seem to want to have it both ways: on the one hand, we're just animals with animal ancestors and we should all be treated equally; on the other hand, we're so superior to animals that we should refrain from acting in the way that they act.

MARIA: Well, again, I don't deny that normal human beings are superior intellectually to animals. Only we have some ability to control our behavior. Perhaps only we have free will, though even that is a very controversial philosophical position.

MARK: So it's wrong for us to eat meat *only because* we could do otherwise, and it's right for animals to eat each other because they can't help it?

MARIA: Yes.

MARK: Sounds like an odd way to distinguish right acts from wrong acts. The same behavior can be right or wrong depending on whether or not the agent has free will?

MARIA: Maybe.

MARK: As we saw with the euthanasia topic, I do think that one's state of mind or intentions can be relevant to determining whether or not an act is wrong. However, this case seems very different and I'm not sure I understand it. Assuming that we really could freely choose not to eat meat, I don't see how that fact makes it wrong to eat meat. Just because we could do otherwise, it doesn't automatically follow that we're morally obligated to do otherwise.

MARIA: No, but we already discussed other reasons why we shouldn't kill animals or eat meat.

MARK: I guess so, but we don't normally hold to the view that "if someone is determined to behave a certain way, then his action isn't wrong." And that's what you seem to be saying on behalf of animals.

MARIA: Well, we do treat mentally disturbed criminals very differently from those we believe to have acted freely.

MARK: Sure, but we never say that the disturbed criminal's act was therefore right. At most, we might lessen a punishment or give a different form of punishment, such as time in a mental hospital.

MARIA: Fine, but it makes the behavior more understandable.

MARK: Sure, but that's not the same as 'morally right.' Understanding what caused someone to do something is a purely psychological and empirical matter, which is very different from making any ethical claims about the behavior.

MARIA: I suppose so.

MARK: And what if human meat eaters said that we're determined to eat meat? After all, even you would have to admit that it's a very difficult habit to break for some people due to early eating habits and traditions. We have all kinds of "mad cravings" for steaks and chicken. So what if a human being, for whatever reasons, is sometimes determined to eat meat? Would it then be right?

MARIA: Let me think about that one, although I'm not sure that we're ever determined to that extent. Anyway, the fact remains that meat eating animals would die if they stopped eating meat because they physically need the animal protein. However, the same isn't true for human animals. We can live perfectly well without the animal protein.

CAROL: Can we get back to the issue of animal suffering?

MARIA: Sure.

CAROL: Since three of us don't believe that animals have a right to life, let's try to look at it from a purely utilitarian point of view.

MARK: Right, we do get a lot of pleasure out of eating meat. It's not just the pure taste of it in general, but also the family traditions, barbecues, and "holiday meals" such as Thanksgiving.

MARIA: I agree that there are, unfortunately, some cultural habits that people just take as normal. And many people find it hard to give up eating meat for these reasons. But doing something out of habit is hardly a moral justification. And, anyway, I just can't believe that so-called "pleasures of taste" can outweigh and justify the horrible treatment of millions of animals every year.

LARRY: I'm not so sure. Calculate all of the suffering of animals raised for food and all of the pleasure gained by humans. Does the former outweigh the latter?

CAROL: Maybe.

MARIA: That's a rather crude and insensitive way to phrase the issue, Larry. But if you insist, then we should get some facts straight. Most people radically underestimate the amount of suffering that animals endure. Meat production is a big business, and helpless animals are treated more like non-feeling machines than as living sentient creatures.

CAROL: Can you give some examples?

MARIA: Sure. Chicken are commonly crowded together in small spaces for prolonged periods of time, unable to walk around or stretch their wings. So naturally they become vicious and even attack each other. To minimize damage, their beaks are painfully cut off. Mutilations are routinely performed; for example, cows are castrated without an anaesthetic mainly because castrated cows put on more weight.

LARRY: And perhaps worst of all is the way that veal calves are treated. I definitely won't eat veal.

CAROL: What exactly happens to them?

LARRY: They spend their lives in small pens that don't even allow them to turn around or lie down comfortably. They can't groom themselves and are denied other natural cravings, such as time with their mothers. The lack of exercise is mainly what yields the "tender" veal meat, since exercise toughens muscles.

MARK: But what if animals could be treated more humanely?

LARRY: As I said before, then eating them wouldn't be wrong.

MARIA: But you still seem to overlook the practical fact that it would be impossible to treat animals decently and still produce meat at quantities anywhere close to satisfying current meat consumption.

And, if it were possible, it would cost so much that only the rich could afford to eat meat. Cruel methods, such as overcrowding, are used because they're the most economical.

LARRY: That may be true. So you think that to work for better treatment of animals would inevitably result in the elimination of relatively inexpensive meat?

MARIA: Right. And, as you pointed out with veal, some of the cruel treatment is essential to the end product itself. So if we treated animals "humanely," then there could be no veal at all.

LARRY: That's fine with me.

MARIA: But, in general, the main problem is that if we think it's wrong to treat animals cruelly in order to obtain perfumes, cosmetics, and shampoos, then it's also wrong for us to treat them cruelly in order to obtain certain foods. In neither case can the pleasure outweigh the suffering, and none of it is necessary in order to live full and healthy lives.

MARK: I'm not sure about that analogy. How you can compare completely unnecessary luxury items to eating meat?

MARIA: Well, in many societies eating meat is considered a "luxury" item. In fact, meat is less necessary than soap and toothpaste and we all seem to agree that using animals to test those products is wrong.

MARK: Fair enough.

MARIA: I think we really need to see the slaughter of animals for food as part of a larger attitude toward nonhuman animals. Innocent and defenseless animals are hunted down "for fun" as part of a vacation. Animals are wrenched from their natural environment for our entertainment in zoos and circuses. They're killed for their skins and their heads are used as wall decorations. It's all part of the attitude that animals are merely things to be used as means to our ends.

CAROL: But some of the animals in zoos and circuses live far better than they otherwise would. And we do also take care of animals as pets. Even you have pets, Maria.

MARIA: I'm just saying that, generally, our society has a poor attitude toward animals. There have been some improvements, but they don't go far enough.

LARRY: Well, let's stop for today. I need to get some rest for my talk in the morning. Remember I'm speaking on capital punishment tomorrow.

MARK: Yes, I'll be there.

MARIA: See you then, Larry. Good night. Pleasant dreams.

CAROL: Good night.

LARRY: Bye.

THE FIFTH DAY

CAPITAL PUNISHMENT

It is the last day of the conference. The scene is a restaurant in the hotel at about six-thirty in the evening. During the day, they agreed to have dinner together before going to a reception in the hotel ballroom for everyone at the conference. They've just ordered their meals.

1. Background and the Law

LARRY: So today is our last day together. I'd really like to discuss capital punishment.

MARK: Me too, especially after hearing your paper this morning. Should we again make sure that we're clear about the law?

LARRY: Of course.

MARIA: It does seem that the majority of Americans today favor capital punishment for certain crimes.

LARRY: I guess so, but as we've seen, the majority may not always be right and a law could be wrong or unethical. Each of us seems to believe that about at least one of our issues.

CAROL: Sure.

MARK: Anyway, I don't think that capital punishment is wrong for some crimes. It's difficult for me to get very concerned about the execution of such criminals.

MARIA: I agree with Mark on this issue.

LARRY: Well, as you know, I oppose capital punishment for many reasons.

CAROL: Me too. I guess we finally agree on something, Larry, although it's difficult for me to understand how you can object to the killing of a murderer but not to the killing of innocent pre-born children. You defend a mass murderer, but not the unborn!

LARRY: Well, murderers are still people and there are also some serious problems with the application of the death penalty. I don't understand how some of you pro-lifers (*pointing to Mark*) can be in favor of the death penalty.

MARK: Why? How can you compare the killing of a serial killer with the killing of an innocent baby? There's no contradiction in my position. It's wrong to kill *innocent* actual or potential people. Remember? Unborn children have done nothing to deserve death.

MARIA: Can we get back to capital punishment?

LARRY: Sure. Anyway, the death penalty has a long history in the United States and in other countries. For example, some people were put to death for crimes ranging from rape to homicide. The situation here is that capital punishment is used in most States, though not very often..

MARIA: And we're talking about *first-degree* murder. Right?

LARRY: Yes, those convicted of *premeditated* or *intentional* murder, but remember that the relevant intention could be formed only shortly before the murder -- it doesn't have to be a killing that was planned for hours or days. Those who do commit the so-called "lesser crimes" of second-degree murder, manslaughter, and rape are no longer sentenced to death. Let's keep in mind, however, that there are hundreds of convicts on death row, and the issues raised are relevant to our entire criminal justice system.

MARIA: That's a key word: justice. It's obviously related to ethics and to what's right or wrong.

CAROL: Of course. Is it true that the death penalty was deemed unconstitutional at one point in our past?

LARRY: Not quite. In *Furman v. Georgia* the 1972 Supreme Court ruled, by a five-to-four vote, that the death penalty was unconstitutional *as it was then administered.* However, they didn't rule that it was unconstitutional *by its very nature.* The main problem was its arbitrary application and the absence of explicit standards for juries to follow. I want to return to this later.

MARK: So they didn't rule that capital punishment violated the Eighth Amendment's prohibition against the infliction of cruel and unusual punishment?

LARRY: Right, but I think they were wrong.

MARIA: The Court basically turned it back to the States to draft less arbitrary and stricter guidelines for imposing the death penalty. Right?

LARRY: Yes, for one thing, in *Gregg v. Georgia*, by a seven-to-two vote, the 1976 Court ruled that the death penalty is constitutional for the crime of murder, so long as there are appropriate safeguards against arbitrary application. There must be explicit standards to guide jury deliberations. States allowed for the automatic appeal of death penalty convictions in order to examine the influence of passion or prejudice. There was also the separation of the guilt part of the trial from the penalty phase. So the guilt of the suspect must first be established and then, in a separate proceeding with the same jury, the penalty would be determined.

MARK: Yes, that seems to be a good idea. And, in the penalty phase, the jury has to find that the so-called "aggravating circumstances" outweigh the "mitigating circumstances" in order to recommend the death sentence.

LARRY: Right.

CAROL: Larry, can you remind us of what some of those circumstances are?

LARRY: Sure, for **aggravating circumstances**, the prosecutor can present evidence such as (a) the murder was committed by an imprisoned or previously convicted defendant, (b) the defendant murdered more than one person, (c) the murder was especially heinous, atrocious, or cruel, (d) the murder was committed while the defendant was evading arrest or escaping from lawful custody, or (e) the murder was committed while the defendant was engaged in other crimes, such as rape, arson, or kidnaping.

MARK: Sound like good reasons for the death penalty to me.

LARRY: But there are also **mitigating circumstances** that can be presented by the defense, such as (a) the defendant had no prior criminal history, (b) the crime was committed while the defendant was under the influence of extreme emotional or mental disturbance, (c) the defendant was only an accomplice in a murder by another person, (d) the young age of the defendant, or (e) the defendant was seriously abused or neglected as a child.

MARIA: I guess we could debate the merits of each of them, but let's just move on for now. I can see how they might make a difference to the degree to which one ought to be punished.

MARK: Me too. For example, I don't think we should be sentencing fifteen or sixteen year old kids to death. And if someone truly has a mental illness or disease, then it seems wrong to execute him. I mean, if it can be demonstrated that a defendant really couldn't have controlled his action, then that should at least be a factor against execution. Of course, this could take us into the whole free will-determinism debate.

CAROL: Sure, but the general issue is: "What is the appropriate or just punishment for certain crimes?"

LARRY: Yes, and even more generally, "Why do we punish at all?" There are two common legal and moral answers to this question.

First, there is **retribution**, which is basically the idea of "payback" based on the principle of retaliation often expressed by an "eye for an eye." The criminal must pay for the crime and is only getting what he deserves.

Second, there is the more future-oriented utilitarian emphasis on the desirable social consequences of punishment, such as rehabilitating a criminal or deterring the criminal from repeating his act and deterring others from engaging in similar acts. Obviously, in the case of capital punishment, rehabilitation doesn't play any part. However, **deterrence** is often cited as a reason in favor of the death penalty.

Their meals arrive. Maria and Larry ordered a vegetarian platter. Carol and Mark ordered a chicken dish with apologies to Maria. They talk briefly about how they at least didn't order any veal.

MARK: Anyway, let's discuss retribution and deterrence separately, to the extent possible.

2. Retribution

LARRY: Great.

MARIA: As you mentioned, Larry, one common argument for the death penalty is retribution. A murderer should get what he deserves for committing such a terrible crime, especially when aggravating circumstances are present. The only appropriate punishment in these cases is death. As long as the murderer is alive, no matter what the conditions, there are always some valuable experiences that he can have. This is not sufficient punishment, since his victim is dead.

CAROL: Sounds like barbaric vengeance to me. I can't believe that we continue to have the death penalty in this country. All other civilized societies have eliminated it. It's simply a barbaric form of revenge. A murderer is still a human being with a right to life, even if he gives up his right *to liberty* and many other privileges.

MARIA: Well, as we've seen, the right to life is not absolute. For example, we all agree that killing in self-defense doesn't violate anyone's right to life.

MARK: Yes. And how seriously can we take a claim of a right to life from a murderer? He denied another person that very right. If a person violates the right to life of another, then that person loses his right to life. If I'm a murderer, then I forfeit my right to life.

LARRY: But even if a murderer loses his right to life, it doesn't follow that we *must* execute him. Does it?

MARIA: I guess not, but it would be morally permissible to do so, especially when aggravating circumstances are present.

CAROL: But shouldn't we be above that kind of barbaric retaliation? Why should we lower ourselves to the level of a murderer and do the same thing to him as he did to someone else?

MARK: Well, we're not doing "the same thing." The murderer unjustifiably killed an innocent person, whereas the government would be killing a convicted murderer. That's a huge difference. You can't compare the two. What an insult to the victim and the victim's family!

CAROL: But a murderer is still a human being. And two wrongs don't make a right.

MARIA: Well, that just begs the question. You're assuming that the death penalty is wrong. But that's what we're arguing about: whether or not the death penalty is morally justifiable.

CAROL: Fine, but I believe that each of us is much more than the worst thing we've done in our lives. I'd hate to be judged solely on the basis of the worst things I've done in my life. By all means, those who commit crimes should be punished, and punished severely, but to take a human life? I don't think so. Only God can be such a final judge.

MARK: Well, isn't there something about "an eye for an eye" in the Bible?

CAROL: Sure, but that's a rather crude reading of those passages. It really only says that God can bring vengeance as He sees fit; not as we see fit. Also, you're forgetting the New Testament's numerous teachings on forgiveness and "loving your enemies," not to mention where Jesus says "he that is without sin among you, let him first cast a stone" at the woman who was caught in adultery.

MARIA: That's fine as a general guide for everyday life, but when it comes to some crimes it's appropriate for a society to hand down the stiffest possible punishment.

LARRY: But I don't even understand the whole concept of so-called "equal" punishment for a crime. I mean, we don't think it's appropriate to rape rapists or to steal from thieves. So why is it appropriate to kill killers? The notion of "an eye for an eye" is really an empty slogan based on revenge and anger. We don't teach our children to act in this way. It solves nothing and only perpetuates violence.

MARK: But murder is a special case, since the most precious thing of all has been taken away from someone; namely, one's life. With other crimes it's also harder to duplicate the end result of the crime and so various lengths of prison time are more appropriate.

LARRY: I agree that the more severe the crime, the more severe the penalty should be. Punishments should run proportional to crimes, but, of course, it doesn't follow that *death* must be the most severe punishment. For example, life without the possibility of parole could be the most severe punishment for murder with lesser sentences for lesser crimes. We should have correlated scales of crimes and punishments, but none of this forces us to have the death penalty.

MARIA: But some murderers don't even serve harsh prison terms, which doesn't seem right for committing murder. Also, the kind of life that some inmates have isn't as bad as it could be. I mean, suppose your spouse or child was murdered and you knew that the murderer was playing ping pong or basketball and lifting weights for part of the day. How would you feel? Is that a just punishment? They can watch television, see their families, joke around, and even have conjugal visits. Is that a just punishment for someone who has taken the life of your loved one? It's absurd. That's why execution is often the only appropriate punishment.

CAROL: Well, I don't think jail is as easy and nice as you make it sound. I've visited a few prisons. They're not pleasant places, and we all know how dangerous they can sometimes be. But, in any case, what kind of message are we sending with capital punishment? We lose a sense of the dignity of all human life.

MARIA: There's nothing dignified about a murderer.

MARK: And I think we can turn your point around on you, Carol.

CAROL: How?

MARK: Well, I'd argue that by imposing the death penalty we're showing the utmost respect for the value and dignity of human life.

CAROL: What? How?

MARK: It's precisely because we value human life so highly that we should enforce the highest possible punishment on those who take another's life. That's the real message: Life is so valuable and precious that if you take an innocent human life, then you may lose yours.

CAROL: I see, but it sounds a bit contradictory.

MARIA: The point is that we're sending a worse message when we only put a murderer in jail for a period of time. Murder someone: get free room and board. Is that the best we can do? And, anyway, execution can even be a merciful punishment compared to what the murder victim might have gone through.

CAROL: How?

MARIA: Well, suppose that a woman is dragged from her car at knife point, beaten and raped repeatedly, tortured with the knife, and then stabbed numerous times. She is dead. Now, you're not going to convince me that giving a murderer sufficient warning of the execution time and then killing him with a painless lethal injection is "equal" to the woman's ordeal. So I don't even buy this idea that the punishment is equal just because the end result is the same. What happened to the woman is far worse. She was innocent, suffered terribly, didn't have a chance to say goodbye to her family and friends, and so on. If we really did punish equal to the crime, we would drag the criminal out of his cell one night without warning and duplicate his crime as closely as possible. The fact that we don't do that is civilized enough as far as

I'm concerned.

MARK: I couldn't agree more.

LARRY: But, again, shouldn't a civilized society try to send the message that even though we are angry and outraged at a murderer for what he did, we will nevertheless control ourselves in a way that he didn't?

MARK: Maybe in some cases we should, but some crimes are so heinous, perhaps involving torture, that it doesn't bother me one bit if the death penalty is imposed.

MARIA: Me either, particularly for multiple murderers or serial killers.

3. Deterrence

MARK: One thing is certain: no executed murderer has ever murdered again! Capital punishment is the ultimate deterrent to the murderer himself. It's the only way to ensure that he'll never kill again. At the least, execution will certainly prevent the murderer from killing again.

CAROL: But wouldn't life without parole also achieve the same result?

MARK: No. He may escape and kill again.

MARIA: Or he might kill another inmate or a prison guard. And if we don't have the death penalty as an option in such a case, then what? What's to deter a murderer from killing again while in prison?

CAROL: Well, it still seems to me that appropriate precautions could be taken. For example, there are maximum security prisons that are virtually escape-proof, and violent criminals can be isolated in ways that would prevent such killings.

MARIA: Maybe, but why take the chance?

MARK: And executing a convicted murderer may also deter other people from committing such heinous crimes.

LARRY: But there is no evidence to suggest that capital punishment is an effective deterrent. First of all, those States which employ the death penalty don't have lower murder rates than those that don't use it. There's no correlation between crime rates and capital punishment.

MARK: Is that right?

LARRY: Absolutely.

MARIA: Maybe that's because so few murderers get the death penalty and because it takes so long for it to be carried out, usually about eight years.

LARRY: Are you suggesting that we execute more criminals? Would we have to execute *all* murderers?

MARIA: I guess not. My point is that if we used the death penalty in a more uniform way so that criminals really knew what the punishment would be, then it would be much more of a deterrent. The problem is that murderers don't really know about the consequences of committing murder. In some middle Eastern countries, such as Saudi Arabia, everyone knows that the death penalty follows a murder conviction. So murder is very rare.

CAROL: I'd prefer that we didn't use their criminal justice system as a model for ours.

MARIA: Fine, but it's a possible solution to violent crime.

LARRY: But you really don't know if the death penalty deters more than, say, life imprisonment. If our society made it clear that stiffer sentences would follow every murder conviction, then that might equally deter murder. Why do you assume that capital punishment would deter *more* than life without parole?

MARIA: For one thing, virtually every criminal on death row prefers life imprisonment to the death penalty. That should mean something in terms of which is more of a deterrent.

CAROL: Maybe when they're consciously faced with such a choice, they prefer life in prison. And maybe everyone would fear death more than a prison term. But I don't believe that a murderer is thinking *entirely* clearly and rationally when committing a crime. I don't think that they're contemplating the possible consequences if they get caught. So I don't see how the possibility that one might face the death penalty would deter more than facing life in prison.

MARIA: I know that I'd be deterred by the death penalty.

CAROL: Sure, but you don't have the mind of a murderer. You can't reach conclusions on the basis of what would deter you, but only on what might or might not deter a potential murderer. As a psychologist, I know that you must appreciate the difference.

MARIA: Sure.

CAROL: And, anyway, can you think of a crime that you *would* commit if you were only facing life in prison, but that you *wouldn't* commit if you faced the death penalty?

MARIA: I guess not.

CAROL: Me either, and that's the point. Although I might fear the death penalty more than life in prison, I can't think of anything the death penalty would deter me from doing that life in prison wouldn't equally deter me from doing.

MARK: But even if we're unsure whether the death penalty is a deterrent, why give the benefit of the doubt to the potential murderer?

LARRY: What do you mean?

MARK: Well, let's assume it's uncertain whether or not executing someone next week in Texas will deter someone else from committing a murder.

LARRY: Yes.

MARK: Why should the uncertainty favor the murderer and his life instead of favoring innocent future murder victims? I mean, if it's a choice between the life of a murderer and the life of another murder victim, why should we be so concerned about the murderer?

LARRY: I guess I don't see how that's the choice, unless you can show in the first place that capital punishment deters more than other punishments. If you can't, then the death penalty becomes unnecessarily excessive.

4. The Option of Life in Prison

MARK: I think part of the problem is that we're talking as if murderers always face very long prison terms. That's just not always true in this country at this time. Murderers are not always sentenced to life without the possibility of parole, or even to forty or fifty years. Maybe if sentences and prison life were tougher, some of us would be less likely to favor the death penalty. But it's so frustrating seeing murderers serving sentences of less than twenty-five years. Talk about a lack of deterrence!

CAROL: But then we should work to enforce tougher sentences or find other ways to prevent crime, not use the death penalty out of fear and frustration. That's what politicians do to sound tough on crime, instead of trying to find real solutions.

MARIA: Well, for retributive reasons, I would still favor capital punishment over life in prison for certain crimes, but part of the problem is a frustration with the criminal justice system itself. I mean, when even Charles Manson and his female followers come up for parole every year, what are we supposed to think? They were originally sentenced to death, but their sentences were later reduced. So you'd think they'd never even have a chance to get out of prison. Wouldn't you?

CAROL: Sure. They shouldn't even come up for parole.

MARK: At least Manson's honest, he just says that he'd kill others if released. He'll probably never get out for that and other reasons, but plenty of other murderers do. It's not even "parole" anymore, it's more like "early release." Parole used to be a small fraction off the end of a sentence for good behavior, but now murderers are freed after serving only half or less of their sentences. It's outrageous.

MARIA: And what about the poor family of the victim? They often have to endure these parole hearings and wonder whether or not the killer will be released.

LARRY: But, again, we should try to fix the system, rather than push for the death penalty.

MARK: But the problem is that we can never really be sure that a murderer will spend the rest of his life behind bars. For one thing, a law can always change or the sentence might be reduced later for some other reason. Who knows? How can we even trust the system to carry out long prison terms even assuming that they're given in the first place?

MARIA: And with all due respect, Larry, you defense lawyers don't always help the situation.

LARRY: Well, we have a job to do and it's not always easy on us personally. No one likes us until you need one of us. But don't forget that I was a prosecutor for a while as well. So I've seen this from both sides of the fence.

MARIA: Fine, but I also wonder about the cost of housing murderers in jail for long periods of time. Why should we spend thirty thousand dollars a year to keep a mass murderer alive?

CAROL: I don't think that cost should matter much when it comes to human life. However, my understanding is that it costs at least a million dollars *more* to have and use the death penalty than it does to keep someone behind bars for, say, thirty years.

MARIA: Why?

LARRY: Several factors, including the additional penalty phase of the trial, the appeals process, and the execution itself.

MARK: But maybe we should streamline the appeals process for economic and other reasons. It's ridiculous allowing four or five appeals. Some States are already limiting death row appeals to two.

CAROL: That sounds good, but there's a very good reason for appeals. It may even be the biggest problem with the death penalty: the possibility of executing an innocent person. The death penalty is final and can't be reversed.

LARRY: Yes, and the system does make serious mistakes. It's very disturbing. In the past twenty years, dozens of death row inmates have been released because they were in fact innocent. I'm not talking about some legal technicality but conclusive proof of innocence, such as new DNA evidence showing that we had the wrong person.

MARK: That is a major concern.

MARIA: Yes, but there are clearly some cases where there's no doubt whatsoever.

CAROL: Well, we disagree for other reasons in those cases, but the point here is that even if only one in one-hundred are innocent, that's too many.

LARRY: And if the appeals process is too limited and if the execution occurs too soon after the crime, then we're that much more likely to execute innocent people. I mean, the innocence of some of those recently released from death row wasn't discovered until seven or eight years later. What if they were executed within five years?

MARK: I think that we should simply be very careful about the guilt of those who are executed. If there's even the slightest doubt, then we should allow for life without the possibility of parole. But there are still many cases where there's no doubt at all.

CAROL: But don't you think it's better for the criminal to have a lifetime behind bars in order to think about what he's done? Perhaps he can save his soul through genuine repentance, and do some good.

MARIA: It's too bad he didn't think about his soul before committing the crime.

CAROL: Of course, but shouldn't he have the chance to redeem himself in God's eyes?

MARIA: Maybe, but why doesn't a death sentence also afford him that opportunity? Of course he'd have less time, but why isn't five to ten years enough time to repent and ask for God's forgiveness?

CAROL: Maybe it would be, but we can't be sure.

MARK: I think that, in some cases, the knowledge that one will be executed might even be the only thing to force a murderer to confront what he did. As you know, unless one is awaiting execution, one will be more likely to deny guilt and hope to get out at some point. Thus, they may never fully face what they've done until they know that the end is near.

LARRY: Perhaps, but they can also have that opportunity when they're old and dying in prison.

MARIA: Maybe, but that assumes that they will be in prison for life. At that point, the crime might be such a distant memory that the criminal may not be able to repent appropriately.

CAROL: I'm not sure about that. But if you think that the criminal would be such a different person after thirty or forty years, then why not release him after that period of time?

MARIA: It may be true that a sixty-year-old convict is literally a different person than the one who committed the crime at, say, twenty-years-old. A person can change significantly over that time. And so it may be true, in some sense, that the older person no longer deserves the punishment because we would be, in effect, punishing a different person. That may even be a good reason for releasing older inmates who've been serving very lengthy sentences. However, I don't see how it's an argument against the death penalty.

CAROL: Why not?

MARIA: Well, if we execute him within five years, then his identity will not have changed very much. So that's all the more reason to execute him as soon after the crime as possible. We won't have to worry about punishing a different person. Those who deserve the death penalty should be executed while they deserve it, not kept in prison to the point where they perhaps no longer deserve it!

CAROL: Interesting. Let me think about that, but I think we'd end up again with the problem of executing the innocent.

They are nearly finished with their meals and the waiter asks them if they wish to order desert. Larry, Carol, and Maria do order desert and it arrives within a few minutes.

MARIA: So what next?

5. Arbitrariness and Discrimination

LARRY: Well, I really still haven't given my main reasons for opposing the death penalty.

MARK: What are they?

LARRY: They have to do with the arbitrary application of the death penalty as well as its discrimination against minorities and the poor. Even though this issue was addressed in *Furman v. Georgia* and *Gregg v. Georgia*, it still hasn't been resolved satisfactorily. I think it's one of the strongest reasons for abolishing the death penalty.

MARIA: How do you mean exactly?

LARRY: Suppose that you had two lists with the first one detailing the crimes of those on death row and the second one detailing the crimes of those murderers not on death row. There would be many crimes on the *second* list that are far worse than some of those on the first. In short, being sentenced to death in still extremely arbitrary, almost random. This seems unfair to those who face the death penalty.

MARIA: But doesn't the current system requiring aggravating circumstances for the death penalty take care of the arbitrariness?

LARRY: It's supposed to, but it really doesn't. I mean, Jeffrey Dahmer didn't receive the death penalty because his State didn't have it, but many poor blacks convicted of a single murder have been executed in other States. Is that fair?

CAROL: Good point, Larry, and prosecutors don't even seek the death penalty against everyone who they believe has committed first-degree murder with aggravating circumstances. Someone has to make that decision in the first place. They didn't seek the death penalty against O.J. Simpson for reasons that had nothing to do with the nature of the crimes. If he were some poor nobody, you can bet they would have. So we must distinguish between the prosecutors who decide to seek the death penalty in the first place and the juries who sentence someone to death after a conviction has occurred. In both places, unfair arbitrariness and discrimination occurs.

MARK: But I don't understand. Are you saying there's a problem with the system as a whole?

LARRY: Yes.

MARK: So why not try to fix it? How is this an argument against the death penalty?

LARRY: Well, it's a matter of justice in general, and I'm not confident that it'll ever be fixed.

MARK: Well, when we discussed euthanasia, you wouldn't agree that since there would likely be serious abuses we shouldn't legalize it. You said we can guard against such abuses and so on. But now you want us to get rid of the death penalty just because there are certain abuses. Why were you so optimistic then and yet are so pessimistic now?

LARRY: Because racism and discrimination are more embedded in this case. And why were you so pessimistic then, and yet so optimistic now?

MARK: I'm not sure, but I didn't say we could eliminate all arbitrariness and discrimination. I still don't see, however, how you've shown that we shouldn't have the death penalty *at all.*

CAROL: Let's try this analogy: Suppose that I'm a teacher and I say that anyone who plagiarizes will fail the course. I discover that three of my students plagiarize papers, but I fail only one student. The other two win my sympathy and I pass them. Is that fair to the student I've failed? No.

LARRY: Exactly. Failing the one student while passing the others would be unfair to the one student.

MARIA: I see the analogy. Some murderers are sentenced to death while others aren't for committing similar crimes.

CAROL: Yes, and this even assumes that there are clear and fair guidelines for when the death penalty is sought, which we've already seen is not quite the case.

MARK: But are you saying that whether a punishment is just or ethical in one case partly depends upon how other similar criminals are punished?

LARRY: Sure.

CAROL: That sounds right. It's a *system* of justice and we can't have selective and arbitrary punishments. The treatment of classes of people is relevant to determining the justice of punishment for an individual.

MARIA: But I disagree. I'd say that the one plagiarizing student *does* deserve to fail the course. It is fair to punish her that way. What's unfair is that *the other two students were not also failed.* Guilt is an individual matter. The plagiarizer doesn't become less guilty or less deserving of punishment just because others have escaped punishment. She still deserves to fail the course. Analogously, no one becomes less guilty or less deserving of the death penalty simply because others are punished more leniently.

MARK: I agree, and even though we should strive for perfect equal justice, it's probably impossible to attain. For one thing, different juries may do different things. That's just the way it is in our system of justice for all kinds of crimes. Criminals are often sentenced differently for similar crimes, depending on the jury or judge.

LARRY: But even assuming that the death penalty is ever just, I'd prefer to have no one sentenced to death as long as others are treated more leniently for the same crimes.

MARIA: So you'd prefer that they *all* get the death penalty as long as the punishment is "equal"?

LARRY: Of course not. I'd prefer that none of them do.

MARIA: But I don't follow. Let's go back to the analogy. Assuming that failure is a just punishment for plagiarizing, wouldn't failing all three students be just?

LARRY: Sure.

MARIA: So then why don't you say the same for all first-degree murderers?

LARRY: Because they all don't deserve the death penalty.

MARIA: But now you're not solely relying on problems with arbitrariness in order to make your argument.

LARRY: Perhaps, but we've already discussed some of the other reasons.

MARIA: Sure, but if the problem is mainly one of *consistency*, we could easily fix it so that even *more* executions occur. For example, we could *require* the death penalty for all those convicted of first-degree murder with at least one aggravating circumstance. But obviously you don't want that either.

LARRY: Right. Part of the reason has to do with what Carol said earlier: arbitrariness and discrimination often occur one step earlier in the process. For example, an initial decision has to be made concerning those we seek the death penalty against.

MARK: Are you saying that prosecutors and district attorneys *purposefully* or *deliberately* act in a discriminatory fashion?

LARRY: Not necessarily. As you know, prejudice can be so deeply rooted in a society or a person that it's not always consciously acted upon. Maybe no one *consciously* decides that race or lack of money will be a factor in seeking the death penalty, but the statistical results are clear. And this knowledge should be relevant when we consider whether or not justice is served.

CAROL: Right. You can't argue with the statistics. For example, only one white person has ever been executed for killing a black in this country, whereas blacks are frequently executed, especially when their victims are white. So there's discrimination not only with respect to the criminal but also with respect to the victim. The chances of execution are by far the greatest when a black kills a white and by far the least when a white kills a black. And perhaps even more disturbing is the economic status of a defendant. Wealthy people can hire better attorneys with greater investigative powers.

MARK: Sure, but let's keep in mind the fact that white murders of blacks occur very infrequently compared to black murders of whites or other blacks. This should be taken into account when drawing conclusions about the relative chances of execution. The statistics can otherwise be rather misleading.

MARIA: Yes, and even though all such problems should be addressed, it doesn't show that those who get the death penalty don't deserve it. It only shows that those who don't get the death penalty should get it more frequently. The same goes for the poor and rich. The problem isn't the punishment for the guilty poor, but rather the lack of punishment for the guilty rich. The punishment of those on death row can still be just. It's the lack of punishment of those who escape the death penalty that might be unjust, just as we said earlier with your plagiarizer example.

LARRY: But suppose you found out over a period of years that a male teacher rarely failed attractive female wealthy plagiarizers, whereas he very frequently failed poor black plagiarizers. Would that be fair? If such a pattern developed, wouldn't those *who failed* have a valid complaint?

MARIA: No. The poor black plagiarizer deserved to fail given the announced standard. However, if one wants to argue that the attractive wealthy females should *also* have failed, then that's fine. But it's wrong to argue that one doesn't deserve to fail because others didn't also fail.

CAROL: Well, I think that doing justice is a bit more complicated than putting blinders on and only looking at an individual's actions.

MARK: Maybe, but we wouldn't ask the teacher *to eliminate* his policy of failing plagiarizers, only that he apply it more consistently with an awareness of any past biases he may have had. Analogously, we shouldn't abolish the death penalty, but only continue to apply it more consistently.

MARIA: And there's one important disanalogy: in the judicial system we have many different prosecutors and juries, whereas in the plagiarizer case there's only one teacher who is the sole decision maker. It's difficult to compare the two since we must account for the differences between district attorneys, juries, and judges across the country. For that reason, we can't expect an unrealistic ideal consistency in punishment. I mean, if a rapist gets ten years in Utah and another rapist gets only five years in New York, does that mean that the Utah rapist was unfairly sentenced?

LARRY: Not necessarily.

MARIA: Exactly. So unless clear specific evidence of discrimination can be discovered against the Utah rapist, who cares whether or not he serves five more years than his New York counterpart? He still deserves it because of what he did. Can you imagine if he tried to argue that he was treated unfairly because other rapists in New York were punished less severely? It's absurd. And, again, one solution would simply be *to increase* the New York rapist's sentence to ten years. Would that make the Utah rapist happier? Of course not.

MARK: Right. If you want to argue that the death penalty is never a just punishment for other reasons, as you did before, that's fine. But I don't see how you can argue that it's wrong in a particular case because others aren't receiving similar punishment. It sounds like an excuse for lowering all sentences. How can it be unjust to punish someone if he deserves the punishment? Why should it matter whether or not other equally deserving criminals are punished equally?

CAROL: Well, as you know, this is not our only reason for opposing the death penalty. However, the notion of *equality* is still an important feature of justice.

LARRY: Right. It's the difference between *noncomparative* justice and *comparative* justice. And what's the right or just punishment can depend on how others are treated. I think it's partly a comparative matter.

MARIA: No. The justice of punishments depends on individual guilt alone. If some criminals are getting away with unjust lesser punishments, we should fix it by making sure that they're also punished harshly, not by lowering the punishment on those who are sentenced justly.

MARK: Right, and if *equal justice* is too idealistic, then I'd prefer *unequal justice* to *equal injustice*. That is, I'd prefer some murderers get the punishment they deserve even if all of them don't, instead of no murderer getting the punishment he deserves.

CAROL: But something is wrong when almost half of those on death row are black while they only comprise twelve percent of the population.

MARK: Perhaps, but there's a disproportionate number of blacks on death row because they commit a disproportionate number of capital crimes. At any given time in our history, there will be one class of people with more of a percentage of their race or nationality on death row than can be found in the general population. So what are we supposed to do? Should we have some sort of bizarre reverse form of affirmative action for death row inmates? Should we have quotas? Should we commute death sentences for a few Italians or Irish because there are "too many" of them on death row compared to their percentage in the general population? It's crazy!

CAROL: Maybe, but, first, the percentage difference for blacks is very large and there's a history of racism in their case. And, second, it has just as much to do with economic status as it does with race.

MARIA: But how about gender? Women are rarely sentenced to death. So if ninety-nine percent of those on death row are men and yet they comprise almost half of the general population, should we permit them to argue that they're discriminated against on purely statistical grounds?

CAROL: I guess not, but at least in that case we know that males, with their more aggressive nature, are much more likely to commit murders. That doesn't seem to hold for blacks versus whites, unless you think blacks are *by their nature* somehow more likely to commit murders than whites.

MARK: No, but the fact remains that there are many murderers, such as Ted Bundy, John Wayne Gacy, and Timothy McVeigh, just to name a few, who deserve the death penalty. They're all white and middle-class, so your arguments here don't seem to apply. I guess I don't see how arguing from discrimination and arbitrariness can have any relevance whatsoever to whether or not they should have received the death penalty.

CAROL: Maybe it doesn't apply to them, but that's where our earlier objections against capital punishment could be used.

LARRY: Right. Well, let's just end it here. I want to go to the reception. It should be starting soon.

MARK: Yes, let's go and enjoy the rest of the night.

CAROL: Good idea.

MARIA: Sounds fine to me.

They settle the bill and start walking over to the ballroom area. They promise to keep in much closer touch in the future.

BIBLIOGRAPHICAL ESSAY

There are dozens of excellent introductory and advanced anthologies in both applied and theoretical ethics. Any of them would be a good place to start for further reading. For example, a very good collection of readings in applied ethics, including the four issues addressed in this dialogue, is Thomas A. Mappes and Jane S. Zembaty, eds., *Social Ethics: Morality and Social Policy*, McGraw Hill, 1997. Other general anthologies covering our four topics as well as ethical theory include:

Steven Jay Gold, ed., *Moral Controversies,* Wadsworth, 1993.
Stephen Satris, ed., *Taking Sides: Clashing Views on Controversial Moral Issues,* Dushkin, 1994.
Daniel Bonevac, ed., *Today's Moral Issues,* Mayfield, 1996.
James E. White, ed., *Contemporary Moral Problems,* West, 1997.
Diane M. Wilcox and William Wilcox, eds., *Applied Ethics in American Society*, Harcourt Brace, 1997.

Prometheus Books publishes a very good series of collected essays on contemporary issues in ethics, including *Euthanasia, The Ethics of Abortion, Animal Experimentation,* and *Philosophy of Punishment.* All are edited by Robert M. Baird and Stuart E. Rosenbaum. I have used these books frequently when teaching courses in applied ethics and throughout my work on this dialogue.

The interested reader will, of course, be able to find numerous other related readings simply by looking at the references in any of the above collections of essays. To be more specific, the above anthologies contain the main articles in **ethical theory**, including excerpts from John Stuart Mill's *Utilitarianism* and/or Jeremy Bentham's *The Principles of Morals and Legislation*, and Kant's *Fundamental Principles of the Metaphysics of Morals.* See also Samuel Scheffler, ed., *Consequentialism and its Critics,* Oxford, 1988.

The above anthologies also contain many articles on "God's Command Theory" and the relationship between religion and morality. Concerning ethical relativism, see also Norman Melchert's dialogue entitled *Relativism: Who's to Say?,* Hackett, 1994. For those interested in so-called "virtue ethics," see the relevant essays in Christina Sommers and Fred Sommers, eds., *Vice and Virtue in Everyday Life,* Harcourt Brace, 1997; and Roger Crisp and Michael Slote, eds., *Virtue Ethics*, Oxford, 1997. I decided to restrict chapter one to action-based theories for various reasons, but this should not be taken as suggesting that virtue ethics is an unimportant alternative approach. A teacher using this dialogue may very well wish to use supplementary readings in virtue ethics.

On **euthanasia** and the dispute over the killing/letting die distinction, see Bonnie Steinbock and Alastair Norcross, eds., *Killing and Letting Die,* Fordham University Press, 1994. See also my "The Relevance of Intentions in Morality and Euthanasia," *International Philosophical Quarterly*, 36, 1996, pp. 217-227. The two papers most commonly referenced are James Rachels "Active and Passive Euthanasia," *New England Journal of Medicine*, 292, 1975, pp. 78-80; and Thomas D. Sullivan "Active and Passive Euthanasia: An Impertinent Distinction?" *Human Life Review*, 3, 1977, pp. 40-46. On the Second Day, Larry begins by presenting Rachels' position and Mark takes up Sullivan's response. The discussion proceeds from there.

On the issue of the "Sanctity of Life versus the Quality of Life," see Joseph Fletcher's article of the same name reprinted in the Prometheus collection cited above. On the Principles of Autonomy and Beneficence, see E.W.D. Young's "Assisting Suicide: An Ethical Perspective," reprinted in the Prometheus collection. See also Joel Feinberg's four volume work *Harm to Others* (1984), *Offense to Others* (1985), *Harm to Self* (1986), and *Harmless Wrongdoing* (1988); all published by Oxford University Press.

Mark's position on the slippery slope argument can be found in Stephen Potts' "Objections to the Institutionalisation of Euthanasia," in the Mappes & Zembaty collection. See also J. Gay-Williams "The Wrongfulness of Euthanasia" and D. Alan Shewmon "Active Voluntary Euthanasia: A Needless Pandora's Box" in the Prometheus anthology. For some of the opposing view presented by Larry, see James Rachels' "Euthanasia," in Tom Regan, ed., *Matters of Life and Death*, Random House, 1980, pp. 35-76. A good place to start on assisted suicide is the dispute between Young (cited above) and Gerald Coleman "Assisted Suicide: An Ethical Perspective." Both papers are in the Prometheus anthology.

Concerning **abortion** and the legal issues, see Ian Shapiro, ed., *Abortion: The Supreme Court Decisions*, Hackett, 1995. Larry's position is most closely represented by Michael Tooley's *Abortion and Infanticide*, Oxford, 1983, and Mary Anne Warren "On the Moral and Legal Status of Abortion," originally published in *The Monist*, 57, 1973, pp. 43-61 (and reprinted in most of the above general collections). Probably the most sustained recent book-length pro-life defense in the spirit of Carol's view is Stephen Schwarz's *The Moral Question of Abortion*, Loyola, 1990. See Schwarz's book (especially chapter ten) and also David Reardon *Aborted Women: Silent No More*, Loyola, 1987, for some of Mark and Carol's claims about the physical and psychological damage suffered by women who have had abortions. On the other hand, see Ellen Messer and Kathryn E. May, *Back Rooms*, Prometheus, 1996.

See also Don Marquis "Why Abortion is Immoral," originally published in the *Journal of Philosophy*, 86, 1989, and reprinted in many of the above general anthologies, including the Mappes & Zembaty. The discussion of whether or not the wrongness of abortion entails the wrongness of contraception is partly based on this paper. For more on the related notion of potentiality, see Jim Stone "Why Potentiality Matters," *Canadian Journal of Philosophy*, 17, 1987, pp. 815-830.

Mark's story of the kidnaped person as a defense for abortion in rape cases was intentionally modeled after the "violinist" tale in Judith Jarvis Thomson's well-known "A Defense of Abortion," originally published in *Philosophy and Public Affairs*, 1, 1977, pp. 47-66.

For similar arguments to Mark and Carol on the apparent conflict between "injuring" and "killing" a fetus, see Harry Gensler "An Appeal for Consistency" in the Prometheus collection. On the difference between "absolute" and "relational" fetal value, see Susan Sherwin "Abortion: A Feminist Perspective" in the Mappes & Zembaty collection. For some discussion of Mary and Carol's dispute over the "oppression/feminism" issue, see Sidney Callahan "Abortion and the Sexual Agenda" and Sally Markowitz's "Abortion and Feminism" in the Prometheus anthology.

Other recent books include Louis Pojman and Francis Beckwith, eds., *The Abortion Controversy: A Reader*, Jones and Bartlett, 1994; and Bonnie Steinbock, *Life Before Birth*, Oxford, 1992.

The two philosophers I had in mind in presenting Maria's view on **animal rights** are Peter Singer and Tom Regan. Their main books are *Animal Liberation*, New York Review, 1990; and *The Case for*

Animal Rights, University of California Press, 1983, respectively. See also James Rachels *Created From Animals*, Oxford, 1990. The opposing view on using animals for medical research is perhaps best represented by Carl Cohen "The Case for the Use of Animals in Biomedical Research," which is reprinted in most of the above anthologies. For more on the dispute over "speciesism," see Richard Ryder "Speciesism" and J.A. Gray "In Defense of Speciesism" as found in the Prometheus collection. These articles formed my basis for the debate between, especially, Maria and Mark on this topic.

For more on animal mentality and the psychological differences between humans and animals, see Bernard Rollin, *The Unheeded Cry: Animal Consciousness, Animal Pain and Science*, Oxford, 1989; Donald Griffin, *Animal Minds*, Chicago, 1992; Daisie and Michael Radner, *Animal Consciousness*, Prometheus, 1996. See also my "Brute Experience and the Higher-Order Thought Theory of Consciousness," *Philosophical Papers*, 22, 1993, pp. 51-69.

The distinction between conditional and unconditional vegetarianism can be found in R.G. Frey "Moral Vegetarianism and the Argument from Pain and Suffering" in the Mappes & Zembaty collection. For more on vegetarianism, see John L. Hill, *The Case for Vegetarianism*, Rowman and Littlefield, 1996; and Daniel Dombrowski, *The Philosophy of Vegetarianism*, Massachusetts, 1984.

On the topic of **capital punishment**, the main proponent I had in mind for Mark and Maria is Ernest van den Haag. See, for example, his book length debate with John Conrad in *The Death Penalty: A Debate*, Plenum, 1983. See also Walter Berns, *For Capital Punishment*, Basic Books, 1979; and Igor Primoratz *Justifying Legal Punishment*, Humanities, 1989. The main opponents of capital punishment reflecting Carol and Larry's views include Stephen Nathanson, Hugo Bedau, and Jeffrey Reiman. See, for example, the articles by Nathanson and Reiman along with van den Haag's reply in *Philosophy and Public Affairs*, 14, 1985; which are reprinted in the Prometheus book. See also Bedau's "Capital Punishment" in Tom Regan, ed., *Matters of Life and Death*, McGraw Hill, 1993.

ABOUT THE AUTHOR

Rocco J. Gennaro is Associate Professor of Philosophy at Indiana State University in Terre Haute. He received his Ph.D. from Syracuse University in 1991. He has co-edited an anthology entitled *New Essays on the Rationalists* (Oxford University Press, 1999) and has written two other books: *Consciousness and Self-Consciousness: A Defense of the Higher-Order Thought Theory of Consciousness* (John Benjamins, 1996); and *Mind and Brain: A Dialogue on the Mind-Body Problem* (Hackett, 1996). He has also published journal articles in philosophy of mind, early modern history of philosophy, metaphysics, aesthetics, and applied ethics.

www.ingramcontent.com/pod-product-compliance
Ingram Content Group UK Ltd.
Pitfield, Milton Keynes, MK11 3LW, UK
UKHW040227290926
15471UKWH00001B/42

9 780761 822370